W9-CCO-819

SAFETY-WISE

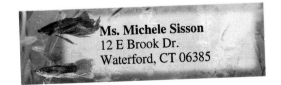
Girl Scouts of the USA

420 Fifth Avenue

New York, N.Y. 10018-2798

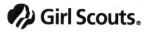
Girl Scouts.

National President
Connie L. Matsui
National Executive Director
Marsha Johnson Evans

Design and Production
Kaeser and Wilson Design Ltd.
Illustrators
Eveline Feldmann Allred, pp. 46, 86, 97, 101, 103, 108, 109, 114, 122;
Richard A. Goldberg, pp. 19, 20, 64, 67; DJ Simison, pp. 77, 82, 83;
Liz Wheaton, pp. 33, 35
Photographers
Peter Brandt, p. 38

Inquiries related to this book should be directed to *Safety-Wise*, Membership and
Program, Girl Scouts of the USA, 420 Fifth Avenue, New York, N.Y. 10018-2798.

The article on pages 19–21, "Oh, It's That Andrea Again! Leading Those
Challenging Girls," by Dr. Sylvia Rimm, is reprinted by permission from *Leader*
magazine (winter 1999). Copyright Girl Scouts of the United States of America.

The section "Finding Accessible Meeting Places" on page 140 in the appendix is
from *Focus on Ability: Serving Girls with Special Needs,* a publication of Girl Scouts
of the USA.

The National Center for Missing & Exploited Children is the source for the
"My Oneline Safety Pledge," on page 130.

© 2000 by Girl Scouts of the United States of America
All rights reserved
First Impression 2000
Printed in the United States of America
ISBN 0 88441 614 3
20   19   18   17   16

CONTENTS

Introduction ▶ ▶ ▶

Today is an exciting time to be a Girl Scout: each girl receives opportunities to develop self-esteem, self-reliance, and leadership and teamwork skills in a fun and safe environment; every volunteer has opportunities to use unique skills, to uncover untapped talents, and to contribute to the community through her or his work with girls.

Girls tell us that Girl Scouting is especially important to them for experiencing feelings of belonging, and for learning values and decision-making, helpfulness, teamwork, leadership, and respect for others.

Volunteers say that they also benefit from their leadership roles. Their responsibilities are personally rewarding and their skills are enhanced. In addition, they gain opportunities to network with adults and to help young girls prepare for the future.

Safety-Wise is addressed to all adults in Girl Scouting, with particular emphasis on those who work directly with girls. It is full of information to enhance your development as a leader, quick tips for working with girls, and lots of advice on creating a safe environment in which to have fun.

Safety-Wise has two objectives: to establish a sound program experience that will protect and maintain the well-being of every Girl Scout by providing Program Standards and safety guidelines for common Girl Scout activities and to provide basic leadership resources for leaders. The leader uses *Safety-Wise* in conjunction with the leaders' guide for the age level of her group.

Chapter 1, "Responsibility for Safety," describes the safety net provided for girls in Girl Scouting. Everyone bears some responsibility: your Girl Scout council, the group leadership, the parents or guardians of girls, and the girls themselves. New safety awards are introduced here to make the point that safety skills are needed for Girl Scout activities as well as at home, in school, and in the community.

Chapter 2, "Group Leadership," will be particularly helpful to new leaders. It provides the keys to understanding Girl Scout terminology and to becoming a successful Girl Scout leader.

Chapter 3, "Group Planning and Budgeting," provides instructions on how to plan a calendar of activities and budget with a group of girls.

Chapter 4, "Basic Safety Guidelines," contains general guidelines that are fundamental to the prudent planning and smooth implementation of most Girl Scout functions.

Chapter 5, "Planning Trips with Girl Scouts," includes preparation, evaluation, transportation, and insurance guidelines and a checklist for travel readiness. New materials emphasize the fun of planning trips and important safety aspects of auto trips. ▼

Chapter 6, "Girl Scout Program Standards," describes the essential components of a quality Girl Scout experience. The standards help adults provide necessary health, safety, and security levels for girls. All Girl Scout adults must be familiar with and adhere to all 35 Girl Scout Program Standards.

Chapter 7 introduces activity checkpoints, the minimum requirements for common Girl Scout activities. The checkpoints are extensions of the basic safety guidelines and Girl Scout Program Standards in the preceding chapters. For activities with no checkpoints, check with your council and read "**Step 1: Universal Checkpoints.**"

There are many new activities in the following chapters that girls love to do, from computers to fishing to wall climbing. **Chapter 8** provides activity checkpoints for camping activities. **Chapters 9 and 10** contain activity checkpoints for land sports and water activities respectively. **Chapter 11** completes the activity checkpoints with a wide variety of other topics.

If you are using this book for the first time, read chapters 1 to 4 and chapter 6 carefully. You can start the process of planning particular activities with girls by reading the three-step process in **Chapter 7**. Terms important to health and safety in Girl Scouting are defined in the glossary.

Terminology Changes

Throughout *Safety-Wise*, the term *leader* applies to the group leader, assistant leader, group coordinator, adult instructor of a workshop or training session for girls, the event or conference director, adult camp personnel, or program consultant.

Similarly, the term *group* applies to gatherings of girls. The same safety guidelines, Program Standards, and activity checkpoints apply to gatherings of Girl Scouts in a variety of settings: all troops and other groups (groups working on interest projects, service projects, or career activities, groups participating in program events or activities in a camp, drop-in center, or program center, etc.) and to girls registered individually.

Throughout *Safety-Wise*, the term *council* may be understood to mean "lone troop committee" for USA Girl Scouts Overseas.

The terminology used to describe all of the Girl Scout insignia worn on girls' uniforms has been categorized for onsistency. A current Insignia Chart can be found on the www.girlscouts.org site under Girl Scout Central, as well as directions for placing insignia on uniforms. The term *insignia* is used for all Girl Scout items worn on the uniform (badges, Try-Its, interest projects, pins, awards, and participation patches). The word *recognitions* (used in former editions) has been replaced by the word *awards*.

All information used in preparing this book is based on current nationally recognized information available at the date of writing; therefore, councils need to keep abreast of new developments and alert leaders to changes.

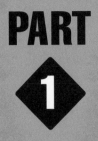

PART

1

Safety and the Girl Scout Group

CHAPTER 1
Responsibility for Safety

As Girl Scout activities keep pace with an ever-changing world, health and safety remain cornerstones of the Girl Scout movement. Safety is planned and practiced by all members. When Girl Scout members learn about safety, more activities are at their command. When participants follow safe practices, they can feel relaxed and confident. While total safety cannot be guaranteed, unnecessary risk can be reduced.

Virtually every type of climate and terrain exists in the United States, and different regions and councils have different geographical characteristics to deal with. To supply safety guidelines for every activity in every circumstance is impossible, and *Safety-Wise* does not claim to do this. *Safety-Wise* offers general guidance that can be applied to specific situations. This guidance takes the form of Girl Scout Program Standards, basic safety guidelines, activity checkpoints, and advice on planning trips with Girl Scouts. The national organization provides this guidance to Girl Scout councils to use in supervising program activities carried out in local groups and at events and camps. Then, through the council self-assessment process, GSUSA reviews the council's compliance with GSUSA standards for health and safety.

Role of the Girl Scout Council

Each Girl Scout council ensures that the Girl Scout program in its jurisdiction is delivered in a reasonably safe and secure environment. The council further provides direction for leaders through training, local guidelines, resources, and advice. In planning and guiding activities, councils may establish local safety guidelines based on the standards included in *Safety-Wise, Safety and Risk Management in Girl Scouting*, and *Safety Management at Girl Scout Sites and Facilities*, as well as the GSUSA guides provided for individual program resources at the different age levels. Each council must consider local needs, geographic or climatic characteristics, and state statutes and local ordinances that may be stricter than the Girl Scout Program Standards and activity checkpoints in this book.

The council provides safety guidance and support to Girl Scout leaders by answering questions, providing training, suggesting resources, interpreting guidelines, selecting and approving sites, and recommending program consultants for special activities. All adult volunteers and

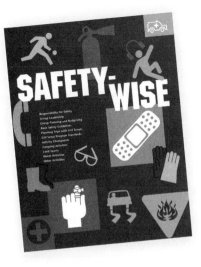

employed staff should know the names, addresses, and telephone numbers of the appropriate people to contact in their Girl Scout council for guidance on safety issues. For USA Girl Scouts Overseas, the local authority responsible for these accountabilities is the lone troop committee, in consultation with the national organization.

The Girl Scout Group Leader

The Girl Scout leader has the most contact with the girls, as well as the most impact on them. The leader sets examples—of both attitudes and actions—that may influence the lives of the girls.

The leader, along with the parents or guardians, is responsible for safeguarding girls' health and for instilling in them the sense of safe living, which is fundamental to their well-being. To accomplish these goals, all leaders must:

- Follow volunteer appointment procedures set by the council.
- Follow all the Girl Scout safety guidelines, Program Standards, and activity checkpoints.
- Follow all guidelines and procedures outlined by the council, including those that supplement or augment GSUSA standards.
- Take appropriate Girl Scout council training.
- Take any additional precautions necessary to avert accidents.
- Be a role model by setting an example for health and safety. That includes:
  - Not smoking. Research has shown the harmful effects of tobacco smoke on both smokers and nonsmokers.
  - Involving girls in safety planning and implementation.
  - Nurturing the concept of safety consciousness at all times, in all places.

The leader is not expected to do all this alone. The council provides guidance and advice, and she may also solicit the help of parents, program consultants, and other local resources. In addition, it is expected that the girls participating in an activity will give cooperation and support.

The role of the leader in providing a healthy and safe Girl Scout environment is twofold:

1. To prevent injury and illness to participants in a Girl Scout activity.

2. To demonstrate concern for the health and welfare of the individuals for whom she is responsible.

Examples of such behaviors are:

- Following local, state, and federal laws and ordinances.

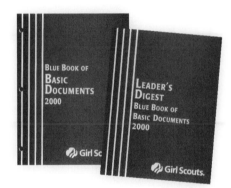

- Adhering to the established Girl Scout policies as outlined in the *Blue Book of Basic Documents* and the *Leader's Digest*.
- Observing the Program Standards, guidelines, and activity checkpoints set forth in *Safety-Wise* and established by the council.

The following behaviors threaten the health and welfare of girls. Adults engaging in such behavior will be released from acting in an official Girl Scout capacity.

- Child abuse. Abuse includes neglect, physical injury, emotional maltreatment including verbal abuse of a child, or sexual abuse. Sexual advances, improper touching, and sexual activity of any kind with girl members is strictly prohibited.

- Abuse of prescription or over-the-counter drugs and use of illegal drugs. Many readily available substances can be harmful if used incorrectly. Since girls can easily obtain many of these, it is important that leaders set an example. Improper drug use can also lead to auto accidents and accidents with activity equipment.

- Use of alcohol. Alcohol is the most abused drug among youth in the United States. Alcohol- and drug-related auto accidents are the leading cause of death among 15- to 24-year-olds. Alcohol is not appropriate at girl activities.

- Carrying firearms. Guns and ammunition are not carried during Girl Scout activities.

Girl Scout councils may have their own policies that further outline a code of behavior to follow in activities with girls, and these are usually covered in basic leader training. If you are unfamiliar with your council's policies or guidelines, contact your local Girl Scout council.

The Parent or Guardian

Each parent or guardian is urged to assist the leader in ensuring the health, safety, and well-being of girls. Parents or guardians should:

- Give permission for their daughter to participate in Girl Scouting and provide additional consent for activities that take place outside the scheduled meeting place, involve overnight travel, require the use of special equipment, or cover sensitive issues.

- Make provisions for their daughter to get to and from meeting places or other designated sites in a timely manner, and inform the leader of any changes in persons designated to drop off and pick up the child.

- Provide their daughter with appropriate clothing and equipment for activities, or contact the leader before the activity to find sources for the necessary clothing and equipment.

- Follow Girl Scout safety guidelines and standards and encourage their children to do the same. That includes reinforcing the concept of safety consciousness at home and in family activities.

- Assist the leaders in planning and carrying out safe program activities.

- Participate in parent and guardian meetings.

- Assist the leaders when their daughter has special needs or disabilities.

The Girl

Girls who learn about and practice safe and healthy behaviors now are more likely to establish lifelong habits of safety consciousness. Each Girl Scout should:

- Assist the leader in planning for safety.

- Listen to and follow instructions and suggestions.

- Learn and practice safety skills.

- Learn to "Think Safety" at all times and to "Be Prepared."

- Identify and evaluate situations where a safety risk is involved.

- Know how, when, and where to get help when needed.

Every girl is an important link and every girl makes a difference.

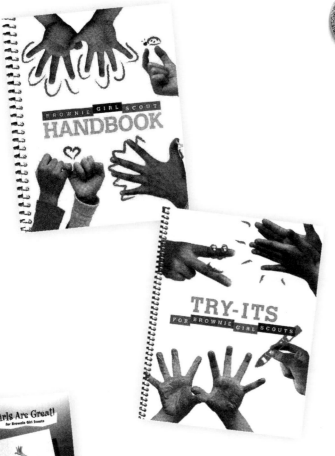

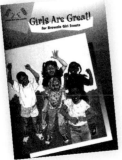

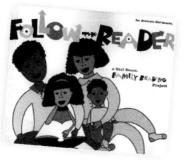

Safety Awards

Girl Scout groups may earn the following awards by completing the required number of activities. These activities reinforce the importance of safety in everyday life and in everything we do in Girl Scouting. Also check the Lifesaving Awards on page 148. You may photocopy the following awards and distribute them to the girls in your group.

Safety Award for Brownie Girl Scouts

Complete six activities that show how to be safe when:

- At home (for example, in the kitchen, while playing, when around pets)
- At the playground
- Playing a sport or riding a bike
- Taking a trip with your group
- Doing outdoor activities
- Traveling in a vehicle
- Using a computer online
- Approached by a stranger
- Someone tries to hurt you with words or actions
- Encountering a strange dog or a wild animal

Safety Award for Junior Girl Scouts

Complete eight activities that show you know how to:

- Inspect your meeting place for safety hazards and find ways to make things as safe as possible.
- Call 911 or the emergency service in your area. Role-play what you would say and do to report an emergency in your home or meeting place.
- Conduct an emergency evacuation drill of your meeting place.
- Give first aid for a cut, burn, and sprain.
- Treat a child who is choking.
- Give a reaching assist to someone in the water from the deck of a pool, a dock, or the shoreline.
- Prepare for a type of storm or natural disaster that might happen in your area.
- Read weather signs to tell when you should go indoors (types of clouds, wind shift, thunder, etc.).
- Check out the safety features of a car that will be used for a group trip.
- Use the trip planning materials on page 45 to plan a group trip.
- Choose appropriate toys and make a room safe for a young child.
- Care for yourself and your friends if you are approached by a stranger in a public place.
- Prepare for three favorite Girl Scout activities by choosing the clothing and equipment and using them correctly.
- Help people who disagree to resolve a problem.

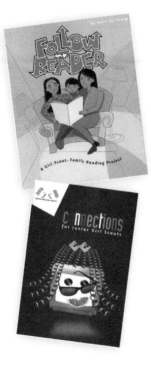

Safety Award for Girl Members 11 years of age and older

Complete three activities from the following list:

- Make a list of your safety responsibilities when you perform your duties as a Program Aide, Leader-in-Training (LIT), or Counselor-in-Training (CIT), or as a babysitter. Create a card to carry with you as a reminder of these responsibilities. Describe how you carried out your responsibilities.
- Create a home safety plan with members of your family. Look for all types of hazards—electrical, mechanical, chemical, physical— and determine how you can make your home as safe as possible. For example, test your smoke alarms and change their batteries on a regular basis. Practice a family evacuation plan.
- Pick a safety topic of interest to your group—for example, personal safety, domestic violence, sexual abuse, date rape, use of drugs and alcohol by teens, safety in a crowd, teen driving and passenger safety. Hold a conference or a forum on the safety issues involved. Create a personal responsibility statement for yourself and your behavior.

◆ Pick a sport or outdoor activity that you enjoy. Analyze all the risks involved in participating in it. Find out how rules, training, and safety equipment are designed for player protection during this activity. In addition, discuss with your group why people like to participate in activities that contain an element of risk. Can you discover why some people seek out risky activities and others fear them?

◆ Plan and conduct a lesson for younger children on how to be safe around pools and bodies of water. Demonstrate the use of personal flotation devices (PFDs) and reaching assists and how to call for help in an emergency.

◆ Take a course in babysitting or first aid and CPR from the American Red Cross, the National Safety Council, or a similar organization.

◆ Conduct a lesson for a group of younger Girl Scouts on safety on the Internet. Include the Girl Scout Online Safety Pledge. (See page 130.) Talk about why each part of the pledge is important for a girl's personal safety.

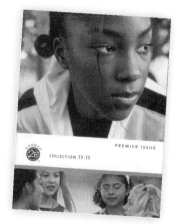

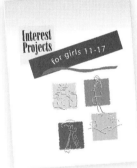

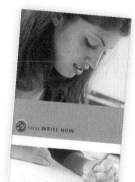

CHAPTER 2
Group Leadership

The leader/advisor is of great importance to the group of girls with whom she works. She sets the tone for the group, keeps things organized, and helps to create the fun. It is a big and very rewarding job. This chapter provides hints for the new leader/advisor on some effective ways for adults to work with girls in Girl Scouting.

When you first agreed to be a leader/advisor for a Girl Scout group, many thoughts may have crossed your mind, such as "What do I do?" or "Will I ever learn all I need to know about the Girl Scout program?" "What will the girls be like?" "Will they like me?" "Will I be able to share some of what I know with them?" "Will I be able to help them become better people because of their Girl Scout membership?" These questions strike at the very core of effective leadership—using activities as a means of helping girls grow strong.

What Is Leadership?

Leadership of a Girl Scout group means mentoring girls, understanding them, and being willing to work toward their growth and development. It includes many things.

Leadership is knowing. Girl Scout leaders are not expected to know everything the girls might ever want to learn. You can explore and learn many things along with the girls, and you can call in outside help for special skills. However, you do have knowledge to share and you can kindle the girls' interest and help them reach beyond themselves. The leaders'/advisors' guide and the handbook for the age level of your group are important companions to *Safety-Wise*. Also, take the training provided by your Girl Scout council.

Leadership is teaching. In your Girl Scout training, you will learn how to break down an activity into simple components and teach them one at a time. Role modeling your skills and values is also a powerful form of teaching. Girls watch the adults around them and learn behavior and attitudes from them.

Leadership is coaching. You are a coach—guiding, questioning, instructing, advising, directly and indirectly. You teach each girl to carry responsibility so that the group will eventually be able to function on its own. The first few meetings of a new group, especially with younger girls, may be adult-inspired, the ideas selected by you and the adults you work with. After this get-acquainted period, however, leadership should be shared with the girls, giving them more and more responsibility.

Leadership is belonging. You are part of the group. As an adult friend, you listen, suggest, support; you contribute ideas, and you help girls implement their ideas. You will discover that the joy in doing things together is even more important than the things you do, that the means are as important as the ends.

The girls will rely on you to provide support and encouragement and to create an atmosphere of fairness and fun. Where would the girls put you on the following continuums after a meeting?

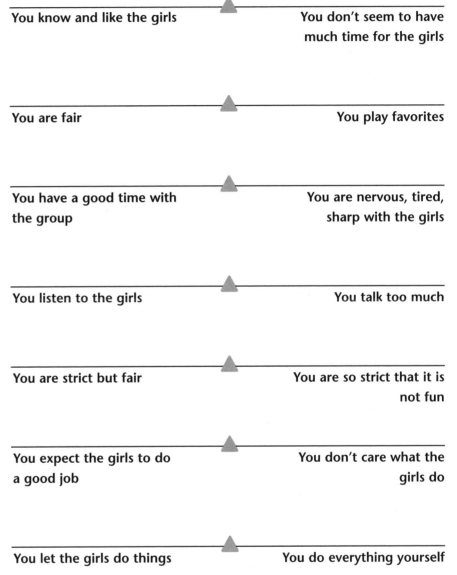

You know and like the girls		You don't seem to have much time for the girls
You are fair		You play favorites
You have a good time with the group		You are nervous, tired, sharp with the girls
You listen to the girls		You talk too much
You are strict but fair		You are so strict that it is not fun
You expect the girls to do a good job		You don't care what the girls do
You let the girls do things		You do everything yourself

What do the girls in your group say about their Girl Scout meetings? Girls have an uncanny ability to spot what is right and what is wrong.

15

Girls expect the following from you:

◆ Acceptance. They each need to feel accepted by you and the group.

◆ Fairness. They will forgive mistakes if they are sure you try to be fair.

◆ Sense of humor. They want you to laugh with them, take disappointments in good grace, and be able to laugh at yourself.

◆ Trust. They need you to believe in them, to be willing to let them try things for themselves.

What a Leader Does

The leader/advisor performs a variety of functions to manage a group of girls and establish working relationships with other adults.

Planning. A group must have a plan if it is to accomplish what it sets out to do. The leader/advisor considers the possibilities in the leaders'/advisors' guide and the handbook, the facilities available at your meeting place and in the surrounding community, and the readiness of the girls. Planning includes giving girls limits to work in, encouraging them to think a little above their present level, and ensuring that each voice will be heard.

The steps of planning include:

1. Advance thinking by the leader/advisor.
2. Discussing ideas with the girls.
3. Sifting the ideas and, together with the girls, creating a plan.
4. Informing interested adults of the group's plan.
5. Putting the plan into effect.
6. Reviewing and evaluating.

Organizing. Divide the girls into workable subgroups (patrols, committees), giving responsibility and authority to other adults and to girls. Spread your attention as evenly as possible. All should feel that you are available to them when they need you. Good organization makes it possible for you to support a girl with special needs, or notice the girl who seems apart from the group—whether because of shyness, anger, fatigue, or another reason. With your adult partners, you can agree on ways to handle these situations. When things are running smoothly, or another adult takes on the supervision, you can turn your attention to a girl who needs it.

Make sure all leaders/advisors, program consultants, group committee members, and other adults assisting with girls know who is responsible to whom and for what.

Motivating. Inspiring girls to reach their full potential is a privilege of leadership. Motivating girls means opening up new fields to the inexperienced, encouraging the shy and timid, prodding the indifferent, and spurring the most capable to even greater efforts. The best motivation comes from within the girls themselves. You set the climate for this motivation by listening actively to the girls, making sure they participate in discussion and analysis of decisions that affect them. In doing this, you will be able to set a direction and a level toward which to strive.

Coordinating. The Girl Scout group is part of the community, a Girl Scout council, and the Girl Scout movement. You can help girls envision the whole gamut of group plans, long-range plans, events, and community activities that are possible. You can gear activities and events to reinforce rather than compete with each other, keeping the whole picture in focus and calling on your service team, the group committee, and girls' parents or guardians for support.

Reviewing. Evaluate what is happening and guide things in the direction they are intended to go. Tools for indicators of effectiveness are found in your leaders'/advisors' guide.

Girl/Adult Relationship

As a Girl Scout leader/advisor, you occupy a privileged spot: you are an adult friend. Let the girls know that you care about them as individuals and understand their ups and downs.

You are also a role model. The girls place trust in you, absorbing your attitudes and standards. Girl Scout meetings must be free of abuse or harassment—among girls, between adults and girls, or from outsiders. You ensure that this is the case.

Safety First

Leaders/advisors must do everything possible to ensure the health and safety of the girls at all times. *Safety-Wise* guides you in planning and carrying out common Girl Scout activities. Some activities will require adults trained or certified in a particular field. In the activity checkpoints chapters you will find sound guidance for avoiding risk when you conduct activities. Keep in mind that participants may not understand the risks involved in a particular activity. Part of teaching a new activity is explaining the importance of following rules and instructions to ensure safety.

Working with Other Adults

When several adults work with a group, the responsibilities of each must be clearly understood. The leader and assistant leader/advisor should be a cooperative working team, each contributing her strengths and complementing the other. However, one person must be entrusted with making final decisions when necessary. This person is responsible for certain business matters, is listed as the leader, and is the contact person for the group.

The leaders/advisors share the job of leading the group and keep in touch with each other outside of the meeting time. It is crucial that the adults trust each other, present a unified picture to the girls, and avoid disagreement or lack of coordination during meetings. Differences between adults should be settled outside of group meetings; sometimes a third person (preferably the one you report to in your council) can add objectivity.

Program Consultants

A program consultant helps with special skills or activities.

Program consultants are recruited to provide enrichment activities and share specialized skills. They should:

- Possess technical competence
- Follow Girl Scout program goals and practices

- Cooperate with the leader/advisor in carrying out the project
- Be appropriate role models for girls

The leader/advisor briefs the consultant on:

- Girl Scout Program Standards and Program Goals
- Basic safety and security guidelines
- Girls and their abilities, as well as on ongoing group plans

Talk with the prospective consultant in advance. Describe the Girl Scout program, outlining what the girls have done to date, what they want to learn now, and in what context they are learning about the subject. Find out what equipment or facilities the consultant will need, and decide who will provide them. Be clear about time frames and stick to them. Be on hand to help when needed, and ensure that basic Girl Scout standards and group safety are maintained.

Conflict Resolution

Conflicts will occur occasionally. Girls may become bored, restless, or tired, or they may be having a problem at home or at school. Sometimes, they may disagree over values and goals. Conflicts can become larger or smaller. They will become smaller if the problem is recognized and if the focus is kept on the problem and problem solving. The aim is to discover a solution in which both participants win.

Conflict resolution techniques work well if the girls trust each other, trust you, and have positive self-esteem. The techniques may be harder to apply if the girls are competitive and rude to each other. If this is the case, you will need to work on the meeting atmosphere. Keep the girls busy choosing and doing activities while you work on changing the atmosphere. Many activities in the handbooks and in other Girl Scout resources help girls build self-esteem and respect for others.

Here are some techniques for resolving conflicts.

Mediation. Each girl tells her side of the story—what the problem was and what happened—without interruption. Each girl tries to develop possible solutions. The girls try to choose one.

Active listening. You or one of the girls restates or paraphrases what each of the girls involved in the conflict has said. Use phrases such as "It sounds like you said…." or ""You are saying…." or "Do you mean…?" or whatever sounds most natural. These phrases can help you discover the main reason for the conflict so that you can resolve it quickly.

Time out. When you know the girls are capable of solving the problem themselves, you ask them to go off by themselves for a set period of time and to return to you with their solution.

Role reversal. Each girl describes the conflict as if she were the other person. This can help girls see each other's points of view.

Skillful listening. The way people listen to and speak to each other is also important for resolving conflicts. Do you look at a girl when she is speaking to you? Do you listen actively so that she knows you have heard what she said? After you speak, do you give her a chance to answer you? Do you avoid interrupting her? Do your body language and facial expressions agree with what you are saying? Do the girls know that putdowns are not allowed in group meetings? Positive communication among the girls and between you and the girls is a large step toward avoiding conflicts in your group.

Applying the Girl Scout Law. Ask girls how they can apply the Girl Scout Promise and Law to this situation to resolve the problem.

Discipline

Horseplay, inappropriate use of equipment, and lack of supervision frequently lead to injuries. Therefore, maintaining discipline is always important. Help girls agree on the ways that they are expected to conduct themselves. Have girls come up with their own list of do's and don'ts, with important extras from you.

All adults working with the group must understand that, in addition to physical abuse, verbal abuse, and emotional maltreatment, failing to provide adequate safety measures and supervision to a girl entrusted to their care may be considered child abuse.

Oh! It's That Andrea Again!

Leading Those Challenging Girls

by Dr. Sylvia Rimm

Despite all your idealism, you may sometimes find yourself wishing that Andrea would just drop out of the troop. She comes in late, talks too much, jokes when others are serious, somehow manages to gather a crowd of nice kids around her, and even gets them to leave other kids out. Sometimes she seems mean, yet the girls are influenced by her. When Andrea's at meetings, you feel challenged constantly.

Then there's Molly. You're glad she's in the troop because you know she needs friends. She's shy and often stands by just watching. She seems so solemn that you'd like to hug her to make her feel better. Getting her to participate is like pulling teeth, and you cringe when the indelicate Andrea asks her when she's ever going to learn to talk.

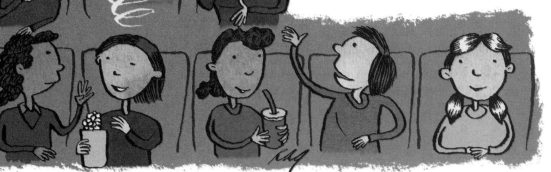

Girls like Andrea and Molly exist in Girl Scout troops everywhere, along with the many other easy-to-manage, well-adjusted girls who participate. But what's an overburdened volunteer to do about them?

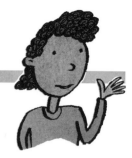

Dominant vs. Dependent

Dominant girls like Andrea actively oppose adults. They're determined to make all the choices. They push limits and refuse to accept "no." They stubbornly claim that you just don't like them, but what they really mean is that they only like those adults who give them special privileges. They seem happiest when they are rebelling or dominating other people. You feel guilty because you know you should like Andrea, but you hesitantly admit to yourself that you just don't.

Molly represents a category of girls called "dependent." They are quiet and pleasant, but hesitant about almost everything. They may get along well with others, but only because they try so hard to fit in. They have little confidence in themselves, fear trying new activities, and are easily overwhelmed. They are usually described as especially sensitive because they are frustrated and cry easily. They attract attention by their minor illnesses, expression, and more requests for help than they truly need. They are vulnerable to being picked on by girls like Andrea.

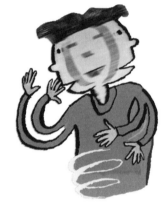

Here are some tips for being an effective leader to all the girls in your troop:

Tips for Coping with Dominant Girls

◆ Don't reprimand a dominant girl in front of the group. She thrives on attention. She'll repeat whatever she gets attention for. When Andrea comes in late, ignore it, but keep track of her tardiness in writing. She'll claim she's hardly ever late.

◆ Quietly and personally praise a dominant girl's good qualities. It will help her to believe she can be a good Girl Scout. When Andrea teases Molly, take her aside and remind her of the Girl Scout Promise and Law. Praise her kindness and creativity in other situations. Encourage her to initiate an idea for including Molly. You might arrange a secret signal with Andrea to let her know that you're noticing her kindness to Molly.

◆ Don't argue with a dominant girl within the group. Tell her you'd be happy to talk to her about the topic right after the meeting. Dominant girls love audiences, and they are at their most defiant when the other girls look on. For example, if Andrea argues about a decision made by the troop, tell her, "That's thoughtful of you, Andrea; I'd like to talk to you about that idea after the meeting." If she does come by after the

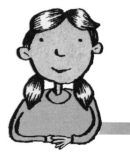

meeting, listen to her point of view, and let her know you'll think about it and get back to her. Tell her that you appreciate her good thinking and that she's taken time to express her point of view.

◆ Be firm and confident. Dominant girls thrive on imposing their power on others. If you're too kind to Andrea, she'll see it as a weakness and walk all over you. If you lose your temper with her, she will fight you. If you're firm and positive, she'll respect you.

Tips for Helping Dependent Girls

◆ Praise a dependent girl only moderately when she does something well. Saying "That was quite creative work" is much better than describing the work as "spectacular" or "brilliant." Dependent girls are easily embarrassed, and high praise puts pressure on them. When Molly asks for help with her craft project, you might make a small suggestion about the next step to take and remark that she's become so independent. Then, let her complete the work on her own.

◆ Pair a dependent girl with another quiet girl for a project or activity. If the other girl is also quiet, Molly will become more courageous; however, if the other girl is too outgoing, Molly may simply let the other girl take over.

◆ If a dependent girl is hesitant about joining an activity, suggest she watch until she's ready. When Molly finally joins in, include her without giving her inclusion special notice, or she'll continue the hesitant pattern. Given time, encouragement, and no special attention, she'll need less and less time before she joins the group.

◆ Give a dependent girl small, specific tasks initially. Increase the size and complexity of her responsibilities very gradually. Big assignments will overwhelm Molly at first.

◆ When girls tease a dependent girl, model assertiveness for her. When Andrea asks Molly when she will ever learn to talk, casually note that Molly expresses herself well when spoken to respectfully. Then go on with the activity and conversation as if nothing was ever said. Molly will quietly appreciate your support.

Tips for Leading All Girls

◆ Stay in an alliance with your girls; help them feel you care about each one.

◆ Praise girls moderately and specifically for their contributions.

◆ Offer personal, confidential comments in order to help girls think you care.

◆ Don't threaten punishments that won't be carried out.

◆ Be firm but kind about rules.

◆ Be a coach, not a judge.

◆ Believe in yourself. You're making an important contribution.

Dr. Sylvia Rimm is a psychologist and directs the Family Achievement Clinic at MetroHealth Medical Center in Cleveland, Ohio. In her latest book, *See Jane Win: The Rimm Report on How 1000 Girls Became Successful Women*, Dr. Rimm found that many of the successful women acknowledged the important and positive influence of Girl Scouting in their childhoods.

Group Planning and Budgeting

Starting the Planning Process

Help girls explore activities in their handbooks and awards books as well as in the many supplementary resources available, such as *Games for Girl Scouts, Ceremonies in Girl Scouting*, and *Outdoor Education in Girl Scouting*. List the girls' suggestions of the things they want to do, help them set priorities, and establish a calendar of activities and events for the year.

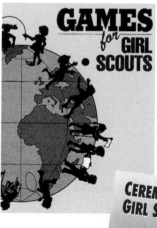

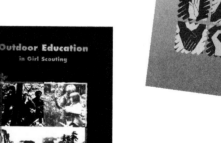

Progression

The Girl Scout program is built on progression. As girls increase their confidence and skills, they can carry out activities that require more planning, take place farther away from home, and utilize special skills and endurance.

Progression is built into the design of the handbooks and awards for each age level. By using these resources and the examples of the types of activities they contain, the leader can steer group planning to age-appropriate activities. For example, chapter 5, "Planning Trips with Girl Scouts," outlines an appropriate progression of trips for girls from Daisy Girl Scouts to our oldest girl members.

Many skills learned in Girl Scouting become the foundation for later learning, recreation, and professional activities. Exposing girls to these activities in their early days in Girl Scouting will allow them to develop the skills for greater fun and challenge later on. For example:

◆ Learning to swim is the gateway to many activities on the water, from canoeing to water skiing.

◆ Learning the basic skills of sports through participation in *GirlSports Basics* is an ideal foundation for all physical activities.

◆ Learning to work with others to plan group activities can foster strong leadership skills.

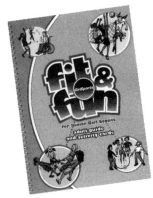

Girl/Adult Partnership

A key ingredient in Girl Scouting is the partnership of girls and adults working together to plan and carry out the Girl Scout program. With girl/adult planning, girls feel involved and have more opportunities to become responsible and self-reliant. They learn how to plan and make decisions democratically, and they develop leadership and interpersonal skills. They also experience a variety of leadership roles in a nonthreatening environment.

Girls need to make choices and plans to mature and develop their competence and self-esteem. Girls who are encouraged to be actively involved, who develop leadership skills, and who accept responsibility are more likely to enjoy their Girl Scout activities and to stay with them longer. The girl/adult partnership begins at the Daisy Girl Scout age level and changes and matures as the girls grow older and gain experience in making and carrying out their own decisions.

Active listening is one of the most important skills the leader/advisor can use to foster an atmosphere in which the girl/adult partnership and planning thrive. In most group meetings, girls should generate most of the conversation and ideas. However, the level of planning and authority assumed by the leader and the girls is not always constant. The leader/advisor takes on a stronger leadership role when safety is a concern or when the girls are trying an activity for the first time.

Leaders'/Advisors' Role in Planning

STEPS	FOR DAISY GROUPS	FOR BROWNIE GROUPS
1 **Do advance planning.**	▸ Select activities from the *Leaders' Guide for Daisy Girl Scouts.* ▸ Evaluate ideas in relation to girls' interests and resources available.	▸ Select activities from the *Brownie Girl Scout Handbook* that will give girls a sense of immediate achievement. ▸ Evaluate ideas in relation to season, meeting place, and resources. ▸ Weigh these ideas against what you know of the girls' previous experiences. ▸ Dream a little about the possibilities and work out some alternative plans.
2 **Ask the girls.**	▸ Give an example and then go around the circle having each girl give one idea. Keep the focus on this meeting and the next.	▸ As you go around the circle, have each girl give one idea. Then call on those girls who are bursting with more ideas. Provide opportunities for girls to browse through their handbooks.
3 **Sift ideas.** **Create a plan.**	▸ Select ideas and make a concrete plan. Plan for safety. ▸ Break the activities into small steps. ▸ Create a chart of pictures showing the plan for the meeting.	▸ Take the most obviously popular ideas. Combine some of the simpler ones. ▸ Pick up on something you can start immediately or at the next meeting. ▸ Put the other ideas in a Brownie Girl Scout "dream box" for future use. ▸ Complete the refining process and take the plan back to the group for reaction and approval.
4 **Alert other adults.**	▸ Communicate to parents or guardians the plan of the group. Enlist their support and let them know what help you need. ▸ Listen to their reactions and adjust if necessary.	▸ Communicate to parents or guardians the plan of the group. Enlist their support and let them know what help you need. ▸ Listen to their reactions and make adjustments, if necessary.
5 **Use the plan.**	▸ Help girls make the connection between their suggestions and the activity they are doing. ▸ Remind girls to refer to the chart to see what comes next.	▸ Let girls know that the activities they are enjoying are the result of their planning. ▸ Use the plan as a basis of learning to make choices, to test ideas, and to deal with consequences.
6 **Review the plan.**	▸ Remind girls of plans for the meeting and the next steps along the way.	▸ Before going on to a new phase, remind the girls what they have planned and review it with them. ▸ Be ready with a quick change of activity for Brownie Girl Scouts—their attention span is short. They do not always follow through on extended projects.

FOR JUNIOR GIRL SCOUT GROUPS

- Consult the *Junior Girl Scout Handbook* and *Girl Scout Badges and Signs* for ideas; think about facilities, season, sources of supplementary help.
- Consider the girls' needs for enrichment, building Girl Scout experiences, and supplementing other experiences.
- Dream a little about possibilities, but do not work out plan before Step 2.

- Have the girls do a handbook treasure hunt. Then have each member write down some ideas to discuss in patrols. Compile master list in Court of Honor.
- Alert girls to intergroup, council, and community events that may affect their plans.

- Discuss the ideas in a Court of Honor, guiding girls on combining main ideas into major themes for a few months. Have patrols discuss a tentative plan and give suggestions and approval to the Court of Honor.
- Be sure girls understand the nature of any future commitments they make.

- Same as for Brownie Girl Scout group. (See page 24.)
- Use this opportunity to learn of possible service projects for the group's sponsor that relate to girls' plans.

- Be sure girls know it is their plan.
- Help girls see the relationship of thinking ahead, making choices, accepting consequences, and honoring commitments to activities outside the group.

- Before launching into a new phase of the plan, review it.
- Expect some contradictory reactions among Junior Girl Scouts. They often want definite plans and complete flexibility at the same time.
- Urge girls to stick with big commitments; let them adjust details to changing interests.

FOR GIRL MEMBERS 11 YEARS OF AGE AND OLDER

- Read *STUDIO 2B resources* and *Interest Projects for Girl Scouts* 11-17 for an overall view of the possibilities.
- Think about seasonal events and projects in the community that girls might consider and what resources are available.
- Evaluate the girls' experiences in Girl Scouting and elsewhere in relation to their interests and needs.
- Relax and speculate on what the girls will come up with!

- Have girls look through the STUDIO 2B Focus Books, and interest project book and propose as many ideas as possible. Use a group government system to combine lists.
- Mark items that are most appropriate for group events and those for smaller interest groups.
- Alert girls to intergroup, council, and community events for the year.

- Use group government structure to refine plans, allot time for their development, and make a tentative plan for the year. Give girls as much responsibility as they can carry. Experienced girls can chair meetings.

- Same as for Brownie Girl Scout group. (See page 24.)
- Use this opportunity to learn about appropriate cooperative projects with the group's sponsor or other community groups.

- Make girls responsible for using their plan, referring to it, and checking it as they fill in week-to-week details.

- Review the plan periodically with the group and make minor adjustments.
- Be sure that the plan is not too rigid to allow for new and better ideas that come to light during the year.
- Help girls to hold fast to any commitments that affect others outside the group.

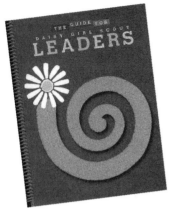

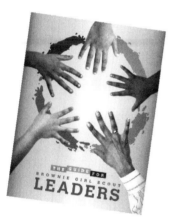

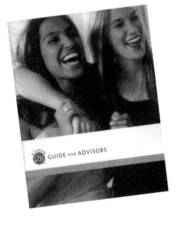

Budget Planning

Group dues can be a source of income for group activities. To avoid constant extra assessment to members, be realistic in determining dues. To establish the dues, determine what portion of anticipated expenses will be covered by dues. Divide this amount by the number of members. This shows each girl's contribution for the year. Determine how many times dues will be paid—every meeting, monthly, four times a year. Do not let payment of dues present a hardship or discourage girls from belonging to the group. The group can adjust dues by cutting expenses, by modifying plans, by more ingenious use of materials, or by adjusting how much income can come from a council-sponsored product sale and a money-earning project. Money earning projects should be approved in advance by the council.

Groups should keep enough money in their bank accounts to cover the activities planned for the year. A group's budget should be based on reasonable dues ($.50 to $2.00 per meeting), council-sponsored product sales activities (cookie sales), and an additional money-earning event if needed. The cookie sale is usually a group's largest source of revenue.

Brownie Girl Scout groups should generally plan activities close to home that can be covered by group budgets. Junior Girl Scout groups may need to plan an extra money-earning project—with approval from the Girl Scout council. Girl Scout groups 11 years of age and older planning community service projects or extended trips may need to plan money-earning projects over more than one year, with council approval for the trip and the money-earning projects that will finance it. Consider putting this money in a special project savings account so that it earns interest.

Progression in Handling Group Finances

Daisy Girl Scouts

◆ Parents, guardians, or group sponsor contributes to the cost of group activities.

◆ Leader/advisor handles the money and keeps financial records.

Brownie Girl Scouts

◆ Girls may pay dues; leader/advisor handles money and keeps records.

◆ Girls discuss cost of supplies needed for activities.

◆ Girls learn to set goals and participate in council-sponsored product sale activities.

◆ Leader/advisor handles group budgeting.

Junior Girl Scouts

◆ Girls and leader /advisor decide on amount of dues. Dues are collected in patrols and recorded by group treasurer.

◆ Girls budget for short-term needs on the basis of plans and income from dues.

◆ Girls set goals and participate in council-sponsored product sale activities.

◆ Leader/advisor retains overall responsibility for long-term budget and records.

Girl Scouts 11 years of age or older

◆ Girls estimate costs based on plans; girls determine amount of dues and money-earning projects.

◆ Girl Scouts 11-14 years of age carry out short-term plans in relation to budget and keep financial records under leader's/advisor's direction.

◆ Girl Scouts 15 years of age and older plan and administer long-term group budget, account for funds, carry out money-earning projects with advice from leader/advisor as needed.

◆ Girls set goals and participate in council-sponsored product sale activities.

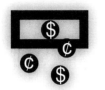

XYZ Girl Scout Council

Annual Budget for Group _____

Date _____through _____

Expenses

National membership dues .... _____

Equipment (new, replacement) .... _____

Materials and supplies (expendable items) .... _____

Trips (transportation, site fees, food) .... _____

Other (food, postage, decorations for ceremonies) .... _____

Cost of money-earning activities .... _____

TOTAL ANTICIPATED EXPENSES .... _____

Income

Surplus from last year (if any).. _____

Group dues anticipated .... _____

Product sales receipts anticipated .... _____

Money-earning receipts anticipated .... _____

TOTAL ANTICIPATED INCOME .... _____

Special Project Savings Account

Savings to date .... _____

Saving budgeted for this year... _____

TOTAL ANTICIPATED SAVINGS .... _____

TOTAL AMOUNT NEEDED BY (date) .... _____

Money-Earning Activities

Choose money-earning activities that have program value for girls and that are consistent with the Program Standards and council policies on money-earning. (See Program Standard 29.) The activities must also comply with state and local laws regulating sales by minors, food handling, etc. Generally, councils restrict the time of year for holding money-earning activities in order not to compete with the Girl Scout Cookie Sale. Check with the council for other guidelines. (Also see the activity checkpoint for "Computers," page 128.)

Examples of money-earning activities that **are not** appropriate for Girl Scout groups are product demonstration parties, raffles, drawings, games of chance, the sale of commercial products (other than those offered during council-sponsored sales), and door-to-door solicitation.

Girl Scout groups and individuals must have permission from an authorized council representative before asking organizations, businesses, corporations, foundations, or individuals for financial or in-kind gifts.

Financial Assistance

Girl Scouting is open to all girls and adults regardless of their ability to pay. To encourage participation, councils budget money to help girls and adults who need financial assistance in order to participate in Girl Scouting. Check with your council to find out what support it offers.

Group Sponsorship

Sponsors help the Girl Scout council ensure that all girls in the community have an opportunity to participate in Girl Scouting. Consult your council for information on working with a sponsor. Council staff can give you guidance on the availability of sponsors, recruiting responsibility, and any council policies or practices that must be followed. Community organizations, businesses, or individuals can be sponsors and may provide group meeting places, volunteer time, activity materials, equipment, or financial support for Girl Scout groups.

If your group has a sponsor, your sponsor's contribution can be recognized by sending thank-you cards composed by the girls, inviting the sponsor to a meeting or court of awards, or working together on a service project.

Transfer of Responsibility

Check with your council about how group supplies, financial records, and bank account information are transferred to a new leader of an established group. If a group disbands, the girls should be involved in deciding what to do with the group's funds. They may wish to donate them to the council for use by other girls and groups. In any case, the funds **do not** become the property of any individual, girl or adult.

CHAPTER 4
Basic Safety Guidelines

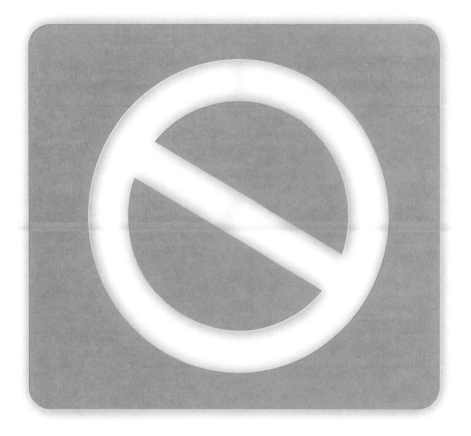

Accidents and incidents (near misses) are more likely to happen when safety precautions are overlooked. Both adults and girls should develop a safety consciousness. Safety instruction, good supervision, maintenance of safe surroundings and good planning can prevent accidents and incidents. Skill, good judgment, and quick action are important aspects of safety.

Good Judgment

Good judgment and common sense often dictate what is a safe and appropriate activity. What is safe in one set of circumstances may not be classified as safe in another set of circumstances. For example, changing weather conditions call for you to assess a situation and possibly discontinue an activity. If you are uncertain about the safety of an activity, give the council full details and don't proceed without council approval.

The safety of the girls is your most important consideration. Because of their youth and inexperience, children need guidance and support from adults. Adults must determine the degree of care required according to the child's age and skill and the nature of the activity. Err on the side of caution when considering whether to proceed with an activity.

Supervision of Girls

Adults other than leaders/advisors who agree to accompany a group on a trip must be willing to supervise the group and the individual girls.

◆ Establish who is in charge. Share your expectations of the chaperones with them. (For example, they should come rested and be ready to help when needed.) Agree on the rules for adult behavior in advance. Establish how adults can contribute their special expertise.

- Provide chaperones with the understanding that the girls have planned the trip and need the freedom to carry it out. The girls know their responsibilities and what to do (from the kaper chart, schedules, etc.). However, girl initiative needs to be balanced with adult guidance, particularly if the girls are inexperienced and unaware of potential safety hazards.

- Anticipate incidents and prevent accidents wherever possible. Review with the chaperones site rules and the rules established by the group for its behavior. Establish procedures to follow in case of an accident; review site and council emergency plans.

Understand the age-level characteristics of the group. In general:

- Let girls act for themselves unless they are endangering themselves or others.

- Be patient. Listen, ask questions, and help to solve problems.

- Know the discipline plan.

- If your own daughter is a member, know how to deal with her in a way that allows her to feel that she is part of the group.

Adults may be assigned responsibility for specific groups of girls or activities during a trip. Establish ways to keep track of group members: for example, count heads, use the buddy system, have a sign in/out system for girls who are going to other parts of the site. Let girls know where they can find an adult to help them during each activity and at night if needed.

Establishing Documented Experience

A certified instructor or one with documented experience in a particular activity is required for most aquatic activities and for certain activities that demand specialized skills, equipment, and supervision. The following list provides some guidance on how to develop proper documentation for equivalent training/experience and determining competence of leadership:

- Course requirements that match those specifically listed in *Safety-Wise*

- Performance reviews from prior

employers, mentors, and/or the council

- Prior work experience including dates and job descriptions

- Results of training/testing/review provided by certified staff with proper documentation

- Grades in appropriate courses (with course contents attached)

- References from people with documentation indicating that they are competent to make statement(s) about the applicant's competence

- Certified translations of certificates/references in languages not understood by the supervisor

Council Procedures for Handling Serious Accidents, Major Emergencies, or Fatalities

Girl Scout leaders/advisors must observe council procedures for handling serious accidents, emergencies, or fatalities. At the scene of an accident, first provide all possible care for the sick or injured. Follow pre-established council procedures for obtaining medical assistance and reporting the emergency. To do this, the leader must always have on hand the names and telephone numbers of the council representative, parents and guardians, and local emergency services such as the police or a rescue squad. Many councils provide emergency contact information on a small card for easy reference.

After receiving the report, the council representative will immediately arrange for additional assistance (if needed) at the scene of the accident. She or he will also notify custodial parents or guardians and other appropriate persons.

In the event of a fatality or other serious accident, notify the police. A responsible person should remain at the scene. In the case of a fatality, do not disturb the victim or surroundings. Follow police instructions. Do not share information about the accident with anyone but the police, the council's and volunteers' (if applicable) insurance representatives, and legal counsel.

Emergency Medical Care

If a minor needs emergency medical care as the result of an accident or injury, first contact an emergency medical service and then follow council procedures for incidents and accidents. Knowledge of and adherence to these procedures is critical, especially with regard to notifying custodial parent(s) or a guardian. If the media are involved, only the council-designated person should discuss the incident with these representatives.

Advance emergency release forms from the custodial parent or guardian (granting permission for a minor's emergency medical care) should be used only if authorized by the council. The council should not solicit advance emergency release forms from the custodial parent(s) or guardians (granting permission for a minor's emergency medical care) without first investigating the laws in the community where the Girl Scout activities are to take place. This step will ensure that such forms are valid there.

The council should also have statements available for parents who object on religious grounds to their daughters' receiving medical care.

Fire Evacuation Procedures

The leader/advisor, assisted by the girls, should design a fire evacuation plan for meeting places used by the group. If a school or other public building is used, follow the facility's established plan after making certain that it will work during the time the group is there. Every girl must know where to go and how to act in case of fire. Consider the following points in designing a fire evacuation plan:

- Draw a floor plan showing all exits and potential escape routes.
- Determine more than one way out in case an escape exit is blocked.
- Designate a meeting place outside.
- Locate a fire alarm box or accessible telephone outside the meeting place.
- Review the plan with the girls. (Walk through the plan with younger girls.)
- Practice the plan with a representative from the local fire department.
- Post the plan in a conspicuous place.
- Conduct fire drills periodically.

Local Emergency and Disaster Procedures

The Girl Scout council should assist leaders/advisors in planning local emergency procedures. Before a place is visited, participants must learn about and be prepared for potential emergencies and disasters. Local emergency management or civil defense departments, American Red Cross disaster committees, safety councils, weather bureaus, park systems, state or U.S. Forest Service, and the U.S. Army Corps of Engineers may assist leaders/advisors, girls, and councils in developing appropriate procedures for their locale.

When a warning of an impending emergency is issued, cancel the activity planned for that area. If an activity is already in progress, take measures to safeguard the girls. To do this, plans for shelter and evacuation from the meeting place, campsites, and all other sites should be known to all, posted, and practiced in advance.

Be prepared for the natural disasters that may occur in the region where an activity will take place. Here are safety rules to follow for extreme weather hazards and disasters such as lightning, winter storms (including blizzards), flash floods, hurricanes, tornadoes, and earthquakes. Review and practice the procedures for seeking shelter and evacuating a site.

Lightning

Be very wary during thunderstorms. Lightning often strikes the tallest object in an area. Seek shelter at the first signs of an impending storm— towering thunderheads, darkening skies, lightning and thunder, and increasing wind.

If indoors, stay away from doors, windows, plumbing, and electrical appliances.

If caught outside during a lightning storm:

- In open flat areas, find the lowest point. Squat low to the ground on the balls of your feet. Place your hands on your knees with your head between them. Make yourself the smallest target possible and minimize your contact with the ground.
- Seek safety inside a car.
- Don't seek shelter under tall, solitary objects, such as trees.
- Don't stand near any tall or metallic object.
- Don't stand in or near any body of water.
- Don't stand in a shallow cave or rock overhang.
- Don't hold a radio, especially one with an antenna.
- Don't hold an umbrella or any other metal object in an open area.

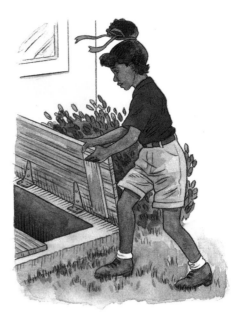

Winter Storms

Winter storms may be minor, or they may be blizzards, heavy snowstorms, or ice storms. When traveling during the winter, take sufficient supplies of food, water, sleeping bags, and blankets to use if stranded away from shelter.

The following steps minimize safety concerns during a winter storm:

- Listen to a local radio station for a storm watch or warning. Have a battery-operated radio available in case of a power failure.
- Check battery-powered equipment, emergency cooking facilities, and other emergency gear.
- Seek shelter and avoid traveling during a severe storm.
- Conserve body heat and energy by avoiding overexertion from walking in the snow.
- Use the buddy system when seeking help.
- Know prevention and first-aid procedures for hypothermia and frostbite.

Floods and Flash Floods

Floods can occur almost anywhere and usually result from heavy or prolonged rain, rapidly melting snow, or dam breakage. Flash floods can occur with little or no warning and are dangerous because of their swift currents and unpredictable nature. The National Weather Service provides flood alerts. Radio broadcasts provide warnings and instructions.

When warnings are issued, evacuate the area swiftly to high ground and seek shelter. Extra food and water, flashlights, and dry clothes will be needed. If evacuation is not possible, determine the best route to high ground. Do not attempt to wade through water higher than knee-deep. Once high ground is reached, wait for rescue parties.

Hurricanes

Follow these safety rules before, during, and after a hurricane:

- Listen for warnings on the radio. Have a battery-operated radio available in case of a power failure.
- Seek shelter indoors, away from windows.
- If you are caught outdoors, drive or walk to the nearest designated shelter, using recommended evacuation routes. Make sure vehicles have gas.
- Leave areas such as campsites that might be affected by the storm, tides, flooding, or falling trees.
- Avoid beaches or other locations that may be swept by tides or storm waves.
- Watch for high water in areas where streams or rivers may flood after heavy rain.
- Board up all windows.
- Store extra water and nonperishable food.
- Use the telephone only for emergencies.
- Do not be fooled by the "eye" of the storm (calm period). Winds from the other direction may soon pick up.
- After the storm, stay away from disaster areas. Watch for dangling electrical wires, undermined roads, flooded low spots, and fires. Move cautiously.

Tornadoes

Darkened skies, thick storm clouds, and strong winds from the south, combined with lightning and periods of rain and hail, often precede a tornado's arrival. If a tornado warning is issued, head for a protected area immediately. Such areas include:

- Storm shelters and basements
- Caves
- Tunnels and underground parking facilities
- Interior corridors and hallways
- Reinforced concrete buildings

Dangerous places to avoid include:

- Cars, house trailers, and parked vehicles
- Tents
- Structures with large, poorly supported roofs
- Gymnasiums and auditoriums
- Indoor areas that are near windows

If caught outside, move away at right angles to the tornado's path. If there is no time to escape, lie flat in a ditch, ravine, culvert, or under a bridge and protect your head.

Earthquakes

Earthquakes generally threaten areas along faults. The greatest danger from an earthquake is falling debris. When faced with an earthquake:

- Keep calm. Don't panic or run.
- If outdoors, get away from buildings, walls, utility poles, and power lines. Head for clear areas.
- If indoors, stand in a doorway or lie under a heavy piece of furniture such as a desk, table, or bed. Stay away from windows. Never run outside; you could be hit by falling debris or come in contact with live wires.
- After an earthquake, don't enter buildings that have not been declared safe by authorities.

Emergency Procedures and First Aid

Emergencies require prompt action and quick judgment. First aid in the first few minutes can mean the difference between life and death. Secure professional medical assistance as soon as possible.

Leaders/advisors should ensure that girls receive proper instruction in how to take care of themselves and others in emergencies. To do this, leaders should help girls:

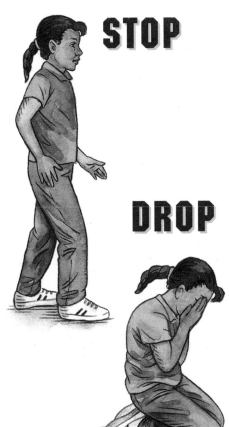

STOP

DROP

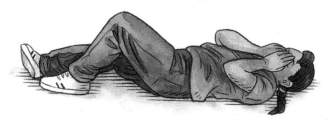

ROLL

- Become familiar with the safety measures outlined in their handbooks, including the buddy system and the three basic steps to take if clothing catches fire:
1. Stop. Running only fans the fire.
2. Drop. Lie flat.
3. Roll. Rolling on the ground helps to smother flames. Or cover the burning clothing with a nonflammable material.

- Develop local emergency procedures that are written out, reviewed, and practiced.
- Learn, plan, and practice administration of emergency care in simple accidents and life-threatening situations.
- Establish and practice fire evacuation, lost person, and security procedures.
- Assemble a well-stocked first-aid kit that is always accessible. (See list on pages 38–39.)
- Know what to report. Understand the importance of reporting accidents, illnesses, or unusual behavior to adults.

Heat Exhaustion

Wear loose, lightweight, light-colored natural fiber clothing to help keep the body cool in hot weather. Drink plenty of water to prevent dehydration. Wear a lightweight head covering to protect the top of the head and shade the eyes. Be familiar with the following signs and symptoms of heat exhaustion:

- Cool and moist skin
- Heavy sweating
- Dilated pupils
- Headache
- Nausea
- Dizziness
- Vomiting
- Body temperature at or near normal

Heatstroke

When the temperature is 80°F or above and the activity calls for physical exertion, be alert for the signs of heatstroke:

- High body temperature
- Red, hot, dry skin
- Progressive loss of consciousness
- Rapid, weak pulse
- Rapid, shallow breathing

Heatstroke is very serious and requires immediate medical attention.

Sunburn

Anyone can get a sunburn, even on a hazy day. Covering arms and legs helps, but burning rays can penetrate light clothing to cause a sunburn. When using sunscreens or sunblocks, be aware of the potential for allergic reactions. Sunglasses, especially those that filter ultraviolet light, are recommended. Remember that reflection from sand or snow increases the potential for sunburn.

Hypothermia

Take precautions to prevent hypothermia in cool and cold weather. Waterproof clothing should be taken along if there is a potential for precipitation. Wet clothing, especially on a cool, windy day, greatly increases the chance of hypothermia. The temperature doesn't have to be below freezing for this potentially fatal condition to occur. Be familiar with the following signs and symptoms of hypothermia:

- Shivering (may be absent in later stages)
- Dizziness
- Numbness
- Dilated pupils
- Apathy
- Loss of consciousness
- Decreasing pulse and breathing rate

Removing any wet clothing and rewarming the body gradually from the inside as well as the outside are important first-aid steps. Seek medical assistance.

Frostbite

Be aware of the signs of frostbite in freezing temperatures: chalky to grayish yellow skin and lack of feeling in the affected area. Warm the frostbitten area gently and don't rub. Seek medical help. If medical help is readily available or the affected area may refreeze, avoid rewarming it.

First-Aid Courses

Throughout this book, the term "first-aider" is used. A Girl Scout first-aider is an adult who has taken Girl Scout council-approved first-aid and CPR training. First-aiders are needed for physically demanding activities and other activities involving a potential for injury. There are two levels of first-aid training for Girl Scouts:

- **LEVEL 1** first aid is required of the adult acting as the primary first-aider for the Girl Scout group activities indicated in the activity checkpoints.

- **LEVEL 2** first aid is required of the adult acting as the first-aider at a resident camp; in core staff and family camping; at day events, overnights, and camping events with more than two hundred participants; and when activity checkpoints indicate that level 2 first aid is needed.

Leaders should take advantage of the first-aid training offered by local chapters of American Red Cross, National Safety Council, EMP America, or equivalent courses as approved by their Girl Scout council.

The following courses may be used to train first-aiders for Girl Scout activities. First-aiders must keep their training up-to-date as required by the sponsoring organization.

The CPR training must be adequate for the participants in the activity covered by the first-aider: for example, child CPR for children younger than eight and adult CPR for older girls and adults.

The following health care providers may also serve as first-aiders for Girl Scout groups at level 1 or level 2: physician, physician's assistant, nurse practitioner, registered nurse, licensed practical nurse, paramedic, military medic, dentist or emergency medical technician.

Courses for First-Aid Training

ORGANIZATION	COURSES FOR FIRST-AIDER, LEVEL 1	COURSES FOR FIRST-AIDER, LEVEL 2
American Red Cross	◆ Community First Aid and Safety including CPR *or* ◆ Standard First Aid including CPR *or* ◆ Child Care (for Daisy Girl Scout leaders) including CPR	◆ Sport Safety Training *or* ◆ Standard First Aid including CPR, plus First Aid, When Help Is Delayed *or* ◆ First Aid Responding to Emergencies *or* ◆ Emergency Response*
American Safety and Health Institute	◆ Basic First Aid plus CPR for the Community and Workplace *or* ◆ Basic Wilderness First Aid plus CPR for the Community and Workplace	CPR Training and one of the following: ◆ Wilderness First Aid ◆ Wilderness First Responder ◆ Wilderness EMT Upgrade*
Emergency First Response	◆ Primary Care (CPR) plus Secondary Care (First Aid) (Valid for 24 months after successful course completion)	
Medic First Aid International Inc. (Formerly EMP America)	◆ Pediatric Medic First Aid, Level 1, including CPR	◆ Pediatric Medic First Aid, Level 2, including CPR *or* ◆ Medic First-Aid Sports Medicine
National Safety Council	◆ Standard First Aid and CPR	◆ Advanced First Aid and CPR *or* ◆ Wilderness First Aid *or* ◆ First Responder*
Stonehearth Open Learning Opportunity (SOLO)		One of the following: ◆ Solo Wilderness Emergency Technician* ◆ Solo Wilderness First Responder* ◆ NOLS Wilderness First Responder* ◆ Solo Wilderness First Aid*
American Heart Association	◆ Heartsaver First Aid and CPR	For CPR training
American Academy of Orthapaedic Surgeons	◆ CPR and First Aid Training	◆ Wilderness First Responder
EMS Safety Services	◆ CPR and First Aid Training *or* ◆ Pediatric CPR and First Aid (for Daisy Girl Scout leaders)	

*These courses far exceed the requirements for Girl Scout first-aiders but may be used. (This chart was updated 1/06).

First-aid training is valuable in Girl Scouting and in home and community life and helps girls expand their safety education. American Red Cross, National Safety Council, EMP America, local rescue squads, and schools offer various first-aid and safety training programs for young people.

In addition, for both girls and adults, courses in advanced first aid, swimming, basic water rescue, lifeguarding, and small-craft safety can help ensure that every experience is the safest possible.

For further information on the training needed to become a first-aider, contact your council office.

First Aid and Infectious Diseases

Many first-aiders are concerned about the possibility of contracting an infectious disease such as hepatitis B or the AIDS virus. To reduce the risks of becoming infected, all first-aid courses teach universal precautions for situations involving blood and other body fluids such as vomit, feces, or urine. These precautions should be taken in all first-aid situations.

1. Wear gloves in every situation involving blood or other body fluids. Keep several pairs of nitrile or vinyl gloves in all first-aid kits.

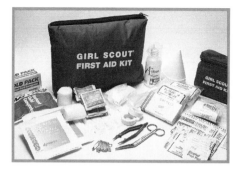

2. Cover open wounds with dressings to prevent the victim and the first-aider from coming in contact with each other's blood.
3. Use plastic wrap or other waterproof materials to form a barrier if latex or vinyl gloves are not available.
4. Use a pocket face mask or face shield with a one-way valve when doing mouth-to-mouth resuscitation. This item should be in all first-aid kits.
5. After giving first aid, immediately wash thoroughly with disinfectant and/or antiseptic soap and water your hands and other skin surfaces that came in contact with body fluids. Wearing gloves, place blood-soaked items or items that came in contact with body fluids in leakproof bags until they can be washed or disposed of. These items should be washed in hot, soapy water. Clean reusable equipment and supplies first with detergent and water and then with a solution of one part chlorine bleach to ten parts water. Rinse well. **Note:** These procedures do not sterilize the equipment or supplies.

First-Aid Kits

A general first-aid kit should be available at the meeting place and accompany the girls on any activity, including transportation to and from an event. In addition to the standard materials, all first-aid kits should contain a copy of a recognized first-aid book, coins or calling cards for telephone calls, and the Girl Scout council and emergency telephone numbers. Girl Scout activity insurance forms, parent consent forms, and health histories should also be included. Before all activities, check the kit to verify that all previously used or expired materials have been replaced.

You may buy the Girl Scout First-Aid Kit (Catalog #15360), a commercial kit, or assemble one yourself. The type, size, and contents of the kit will vary according to where it is to be used—for example, at the meeting place or on a camping trip. Consult a physician for specific recommendations.

Your kit should contain the standard materials in the following list. The purpose for some of the materials is given to ensure that their use is clearly understood.

◆ Adhesive tape and bandages
◆ Alcohol wipes
◆ Band-Aids, assorted sizes
◆ Bottle of distilled water (to use as an eye rinse or to clean wounds or other items)

- Coins for phone calls
- First-aid book
- Flashlight
- Gauze pads
- Instant chemical icepack
- Nitrile or vinyl gloves (disposable, to use in situations involving blood or other body fluids)
- List of emergency phone numbers
- Oral thermometer
- Paper drinking cups
- Plastic bags (to dispose of used materials and to collect vomitus for analysis in suspected oral poisonings)
- Pocket face mask or face shield (to use when performing mouth-to-mouth resuscitation)
- Roller gauze bandages
- Safety pins
- Scissors
- Soap (antibacterial liquid)
- Splints
- Triangular bandages
- Tweezers
- White index cards, transparent tape, and self-closing plastic bag (to use when removing objects such as ticks; tape the removed item to the index card, enclose it in the plastic bag, and give it to the medical professional)

Additional supplies you may need are personal care products (for example, sanitary napkins or tampons).

Medications

Parents or guardians of girls who take prescribed medications (for example, allergy pills) should inform leaders in advance. Over-the-counter or prescribed medications should be in the original container and administered in the prescribed dosage by or in the presence of the responsible adult as per the written instructions of a custodial parent, a guardian, or a physician. Medications, including over-the-counter products, should never be given without prior written permission from a girl's custodial parent or guardian. Some girls may need to carry and administer their own medications, such as bronchial inhalers. Leaders should be notified of such a circumstance as well.

Health Histories/Health Examinations

As noted in the text accompanying Program Standard 3 (page 64), a health history is required annually for participation in physically demanding activities such as water sports, horseback riding, or skiing. A health examination within the preceding 24 months is required for participation in resident camping, in a trip of more than three nights, or in organized competitive sports. A health history or health examination may be required of adults participating in extended *trips* or physically demanding activities.

Information from a health examination is confidential and should only be shared with persons who have a need to know in order to protect the health and safety of the participant and other participants. The statement may include accommodations that are determined to be necessary to allow participation in the activity. If the leader cannot determine how the accommodation(s) may be accomplished, she should ask the council for assistance.

Although health examinations are necessary to protect the health and welfare of the girls, obtaining them may be a financial burden for some. Councils and leaders are urged to explore alternatives for meeting this requirement. For example:

- The health examination may be given by a licensed physician, nurse practitioner, physician's assistant, or registered nurse.
- A girl may obtain a copy of her current school health examination record.
- A girl may use a clinic or community health services, such as the health department, the U.S. Army Medical Corps, or college or university medical schools.
- The council may collaborate with an organization that is willing to sponsor a health examination clinic.

Guidelines for Sensitive Issues

In order to be contemporary and responsive to the girls' needs and interests, some Girl Scout activities focus on subjects that may be considered sensitive or controversial. There is no definitive list of these subjects. In general, highly personal topics such as human sexuality, religious beliefs, and cultural and family values are sensitive. Subjects such as AIDS, child abuse, suicide, and teenage pregnancy are other examples. Good judgment is required since what may be considered sensitive in one part of the country or by one group of people may not be classified the same way in another section of the country or by another group. Many subjects can become controversial if handled inappropriately. Therefore, it is important to follow council procedures for handling sensitive issues.

When Girl Scout program activities involve sensitive or controversial issues, the leader's/advisor's role is as a caring adult who can help girls acquire their own skills and knowledge in a supportive atmosphere rather than as an advocate of any particular position.

Since most sensitive topics are rooted in people's values, parental support and understanding are crucial to the success of all activities on these topics. Involving parents and guardians in the activities that girls do in a group meeting or at home will go far toward reassuring them of the quality and benefits of these activities. (See Program Standard 10, "Parental Permission," on page 67.) Before covering any sensitive issue beyond the scope of the Girl Scout program resources, obtain council support and approval.

Program consultants and special resource consultants are often used to deliver programs on sensitive issues. They should understand and be willing to adhere to Girl Scout national policies and the Girl Scout position on human sexuality and related topics.

When discussing sensitive values issues, encourage girls to talk with resource people, such as family members, religious leaders, and appropriate experts. A girl should hear all sides of a question and be guided by her parents or guardian and her religious teachings before she makes a decision. Encourage the girls to see that each family has its own way of doing things based on family customs, religion, cultural background, lifestyles, and so on. Encourage the girls to try to understand parental decisions by examining their parent's point of view.

Help girls consider the possible consequences of an action they are considering. Girls need to see the importance of weighing future implications of an action against the immediate result.

The Issues for Girl Scouts series does not contain information or activities that are any more sensitive or controversial than what is currently printed in Girl Scout handbooks for each age level. Although leaders should have acquired skills in facilitating program activities and girl planning before introducing these materials, they are not required to have specific training for each topic covered in the Issues for Girl Scouts series. However, when implementing these resources, adults need to be sensitive to the particular values and practices in their communities.

Girl Scouting plays a vital role in helping girls to make informed, responsible decisions about their well-being. Assure the girls of your trust in them and your confidence in their ability to make decisions that are correct for them.

Tips for Handling Specific Sensitive Situations with Girls

If a Girl Scout leader/advisor notices signs of substance abuse, child abuse, suicidal behavior, or eating disorders (anorexia nervosa and bulimia), she should notify her council or follow any established council procedures. Reporting information to people who can help is crucial to protecting children. In some cases, it is also the law.

General tips for how to handle specific sensitive situations follow. More detailed information is included in the Issues for Girl Scouts booklets for the topic discussed.

Substance Abuse

Many young people abuse one or more substances, and many more are being pressured to do so by their peers, media images, etc. Alcohol is the most abused drug among youth in the United States, followed by tobacco.

The following are possible signs of drug involvement. Keep in mind that these signs can also be attributed to other stresses in a girl's life.

- Changes in behavior—including disruptive, delinquent behavior
- A drop in the quality of schoolwork and in grades
- Withdrawal from school and family activities
- Increased secretiveness
- Changes in friendships
- Erratic mood changes, apathy, and lethargy
- Overreacting, overly sensitive responses
- Disappearance of money and other valuables
- Neglect of personal appearance and hygiene

- Presence of drug paraphernalia, incense, room deodorizer, eyedropper bottles, drugs
- Chronic lying
- Physical symptoms such as red eyes, sores on nose or mouth, fatigue, drowsiness, loss or gain in appetite, altered speech, puncture marks on arm
- Sudden constant runny nose
- Eating extremes, unexplained weight loss
- Dulled speech and expression
- Wearing sunglasses unnecessarily
- Avoidance of eye contact
- Problems with concentration and memory

If you notice these signs, follow council guidelines for reporting this information.

Child Abuse

Child abuse affects more than one million children each year in the United States. Physical abuse, sexual abuse, emotional maltreatment, and physical neglect are four common types of abuse.

Many abused children show some of the following symptoms: low self-esteem; anger; guilt; aggressive, hyperactive, or disruptive behavior; withdrawal; delinquent behavior; poor school performance; and abuse of drugs and alcohol. The Issues for Girl Scouts booklet *Staying Safe: Preventing Child Abuse* contains more

specific signs for each type of abuse.

Since child abuse is a crime, there is an agency mandated in every state to receive and investigate reports of suspected child abuse. In some states, Girl Scout leaders are considered to be mandated reporters. Check with your local Girl Scout council to determine your reporting responsibilities.

If a girl says she has been abused:

- Treat what the girl has said as fact.
- Assure her that the abuse is not her fault. Commend her for telling you about it.
- Be sympathetic and nonjudgmental.
- Consult with your council contact to determine appropriate next steps.

Some possible signs of abuse are:

- Unexplained injuries such as bruises, burns, or fractures
- Excessive fearfulness or distrust of adults
- Abusive behavior toward other children, especially younger ones
- Avoidance of physical contact

If you suspect that a girl has been abused but you have not specifically been told about it, do the following:

◆ Consult with your council to determine the appropriate course of action.

◆ Report the suspected abuse to the agency in your state mandated to receive and investigate such cases.

Since abuse can happen in any environment, volunteers and staff who work directly with girls should:

◆ Be familiar with and observe all council guidelines related to preventing child abuse.

◆ Follow adult supervision guidelines outlined in this book and any additional council guidelines to ensure that there is no risk of abuse in the Girl Scout setting.

Suicide

Every year in the United States, more than five thousand young people commit suicide and as many as a half million more attempt it. Suicide is the third-leading cause of death among adolescents.

Take any suicide threat seriously. Talk to a reliable family member or guardian. Notify appropriate council personnel and/or health care professionals.

Be alert to the warning signs of suicide:

◆ Long-standing depression (sometimes manifested as boredom, agi-

tation, acting-out behavior, or physical symptoms such as headaches). Particular danger points are when a girl is going into and apparently recovering from depression.

◆ Previous suicide attempts, suicidal gestures, or verbal suicide threats or other statements indicating a desire to die

◆ Marked changes in behavior or personality (for example, unusual moodiness, aggressiveness, or sensitivity)

◆ Eating and sleep disturbances

◆ Declining academic performance and/or inability to concentrate

◆ Withdrawal from family and friends

◆ Fatigue, apathy, or loss of interest in previously enjoyed activities

◆ Deterioration in appearance and personal hygiene

◆ Giving away prized possessions

◆ Preoccupation with the subject of death

◆ Recent traumatic events, such as the death of a family member

◆ Feelings of worthlessness and hopelessness, of not being loved or appreciated

If a girl seems suicidal or has threatened suicide:

◆ Trust your instincts. Don't ignore the warning signs.

◆ Don't pull away from her. Remember that suicidal adolescents rarely seek professional help on their own.

◆ Don't leave the girl alone if the situation is immediately life-threatening. If necessary, call a responsible family member or even the police.

◆ Be sympathetic. Reassure her that she has someone to turn to and that she can be helped.

◆ Offer to help her, but don't agree to keep information confidential if she reveals something that might affect her safety.

◆ Don't offer reassurances that may not be true.

◆ Speak with your council contact to determine appropriate action.

Eating Disorders

Anorexia nervosa and bulimia are eating disorders characterized by a preoccupation with food, an irrational fear of being fat, and a distorted body image. Anorexia involves a dramatic weight loss due to self-starvation or severe self-imposed dieting. Bulimia involves binge eating and purging accompanied by frequent weight fluctuations, rather than extreme, continuous weight loss. It is estimated that anorexia strikes more than one in every one hundred teenage girls and young women; the rate is much higher for bulimia.

If you suspect that a girl is bulimic or anorexic, try to talk with her about the problem. These disorders can be serious, even life-threatening, so early detection and treatment are crucial. Alert parents or guardians, and contact the council office for sources of professional help. The friendships found in Girl Scouting can be an important adjunct to therapy and should be supported.

AIDS

AIDS stands for Acquired Immune Deficiency Syndrome, a disease in which the body's immune system breaks down. AIDS is caused by human immunodeficiency virus (HIV).

The AIDS virus can be spread through sexual contact with an infected person, using an infected person's unsterilized needles or syringes, blood transfusions prior to 1985, and during pregnancy if the mother is infected. AIDS is not spread by sneezing or coughing or by touching doorknobs, toilets, dishes, clothing, or other things in the home or outside the home.

Since there is a risk of infection when blood and other body fluids are involved, girls and adults should take the precautions outlined on page 38.

If you suspect a girl is HIV positive or has AIDS, follow council procedures for handling such situations. To date, it has been determined that children testing positive for the AIDS virus do not pose a risk to others in a school or social setting. None of the cases of AIDS in the United States are suspected of having been transmitted from one child to another in the home, at school, in foster care, or in a day-care setting. On the contrary, the child whose immune system is damaged by AIDS is highly susceptible to infections from other children in a school or social setting. The child's physician can best assess any risk from participation in Girl Scout group activities. Also, many states have adopted confidentiality laws involving persons with AIDS and HIV. You must respect the privacy of all persons.

Remember, advance knowledge of what to do will help you respond effectively to these sensitive situations.

Service Projects

Girls may not participate in service projects that involve health and safety risks—for example, service projects requiring specialized training or certification, such as lead paint removal.

Service projects involving litter pick-ups, stream cleanup, adopt-a-highway programs, and other such activities that involve girls, adults, and/or families picking up trash to beautify an area, need to be carefully planned because they present the following risks:

- Unless all debris is disposed of properly and completely, the Girl Scout council involved with the cleanup may be held liable for its illegal disposal. Special permission may be obtained by the council through its EPA regional office.
- Having children clean up along highways being used by fast-moving vehicles can present the possibility of a serious accident, unless careful coordination is established with the highway or local police. Roadside cleanups should not be done by Daisy and Brownie Girl Scouts.
- There can be serious disease potential involved in having children pick up trash, which may contain discarded drug needles, medical wastes, etc. Girls should wear gloves and be carefully instructed about the types of items they are to pick up. Special receptacles should be provided for sharp articles so that they do not protrude through a plastic trash bag and cut someone who moves the bag.

CHAPTER 5
Planning Trips with Girl Scouts

A Girl Scout trip is an opportunity for girls to have fun, to experience adventure, and to enrich the ongoing Girl Scout program. Sometimes a trip is the culmination of a progression of activities that the girls are already engaged in.

The Planning Process

Learning how to plan a trip is a progressive experience for a Girl Scout, one that starts with a simple outing. Daisy Girl Scouts, for example, might begin with a discovery walk. Even older girls should start with simple trips if they have never traveled.

Photocopy and cut apart the cards on page 45. Ask the girls to put them in order and then use them to plan a trip.

When the girls understand the planning process, they can progress to longer trips. Whether the trip is a day hike or a cross-country trek, the basic steps are essentially the same.

The details grow as the trip becomes more complex or when the composition of the group changes, but the process is the same.

Every group that plans a trip starts with the same questions:

- Where are we going?
- Why are we going?
- When are we going?
- How will we get there?
- How much will it cost?
- How should we get ready?
- Will everyone be able to go?
- Where is emergency help available?
- What safety factors must we consider?
- What will we do along the way?
- What will we do when we get there?
- What will we do when we return home?

The girls answer all these questions in working out their own trip. Through the planning process, they learn how to develop overall plans, make arrangements, budget and handle money, and accept responsibility for personal conduct and safety. Afterward, they evaluate the experience and share it with others.

▶▶ **Show how to get a vehicle ready for a trip by checking tire pressure and oil, lights, and horn. Are all the seat belts working and windows clean?**

Do a demonstration to show how you would evacuate a vehicle in an emergency and what you would do next.

▶▶ **Map out your route.**

Where will you stop along the way for a break if the drive is more than two hours long?

▶▶ **Plan your trip.**

Where we want to go:

When we will go:

Who will go:

What we will do:

What it will cost:

▶▶ **Check the group's first-aid kit and restock it for your trip, if needed.**

Special needs for this trip:

Plan snacks and beverages to take on your trip.

▶▶ **Do a skit to show how you will walk together at your destination, cross streets as a group, etc.**

▶▶ **Make a list of what to wear and what to pack for your trip.**

What to wear:

What to pack:

▶▶ **What do we need to do to be safe in the vehicle? Example: Wear seat belts, keep arms and heads inside.**

Brainstorm a list of activities to do in the car that will not distract the driver.

Examples:
Alphabet and license plate games.

▶▶ **Which parents or guardians can help?**

Drivers:

Adults to go with us:

First-aider, if needed:

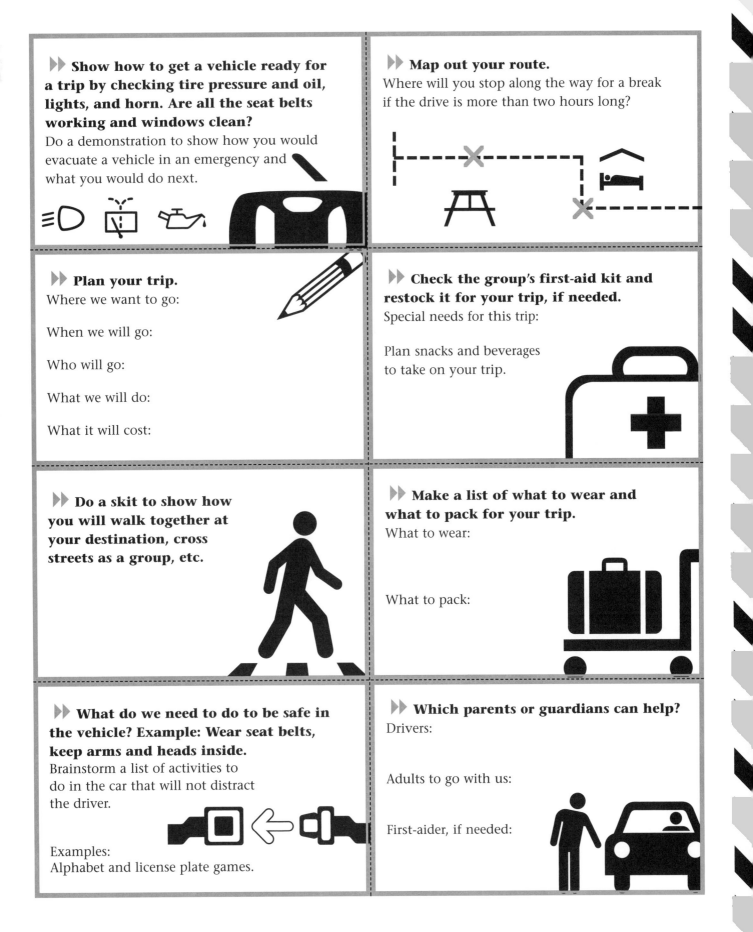

The Progression of Trips

Meeting-time trips to points of interest in the neighborhood—for example, a walk to a nearby garden or a short ride by car or public transportation to the firehouse or the courthouse—are the simplest and start the progression.

Day trips are next. These are daytime excursions away from the group meeting place and outside the regular meeting time. Girls might plan an all-day visit to a point of historical or natural interest, bringing their own lunch. Or they might go to a nearby city, scheduling time for a meal in a restaurant.

Simple overnight trips usually involve one or two nights away. The destination may be a nearby state or national park, historic site, or city for sightseeing. The group may stay in a hostel, hotel, or motel, or they may camp at a Girl Scout campsite or nearby campgrounds.

Extended overnight trips range from three nights or more spent at camp to extensive travel within the continental United States. The group might use several accommodations and modes of transportation throughout the trip. For further information about travel camping facilities at Girl Scout sites across the country, obtain GSUSA's Trekking Network Directory from your council office.

Wider opportunities are Girl Scout activities/experiences that take place outside the group. They can be neighborhood, council, state, national, or international experiences. Wider opportunities with nationwide participation are promoted annually in *Wider Ops*, which is sent to girls 12 years of age and older and to their leaders.

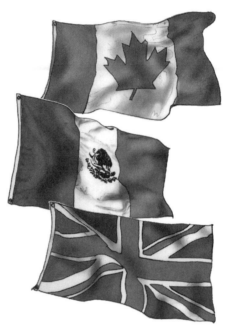

International trips, such as to Canada, Mexico, and England, are available to girls 14 years old and older who have successfully taken overnight trips. Because such trips are subject to special requirements, including regulations and procedures of the World Association of Girl Guides and Girl Scouts (WAGGGS), they are dealt with in a special section on pages 59–60.

Progression by Age Level

Even though girls differ in their abilities and their past experiences, it is possible to make generalizations about trips and travel preparations appropriate to each age level. For each age level, be prepared to make reasonable accommodations so that girls who may have disabilities can participate.

Reminder: Leaders must always obtain council permission for trips.

The leader provides the following information to the council when seeking approval for a given activity:

- An itinerary
- The type of activity and the specific activities involved
- The location and kind of premises that will be used
- Inclusive dates and times
- The number of girls who will be participating. Parental permissions must be obtained.
- The number of adults participating, their gender, and their roles
- The participants' skill level
- Special consultants or resource people who will be involved
- Other groups or organizations that will be involved
- The planned safety precautions
- Specialized equipment that will be used
- The mode of transportation

◆ Specific activities involved

◆ Any required special agreements or contracts (for example, hiring a bus, use of premises)

Daisy Girl Scouts

Daisy Girl Scout travel activities include local field trips (up to a day long) and overnight camping trips with family members. In the Daisy Girl Scout circle, girls can help to choose specific places they would like to go.

Brownie Girl Scouts

Brownie Girl Scouts go on discovery trips in the neighborhood or nearby. The girls may have the idea for taking a trip or a leader or an older Girl Scout may stimulate the discussion. In the Brownie Girl Scout Ring, the girls talk about what they would like to do; the leader helps them narrow their ideas to those that are within their abilities and budget. The girls can then vote on the trip they want to take and on alternative plans.

For travel of any distance, the leader finds out how long the trip will take, checks points of interest to Brownie Girl Scouts, and makes arrangements for places to eat and for rest stops. She sets arrival and departure times, schedules tours, arranges transportation, and obtains the permission of a parent or guardian. Group committee members or older Girl Scouts

may help with these pretrip plans.

Brownie Girl Scouts and their leader talk about what they will see and do on the trip, what they need to bring with them, how much the trip will cost, and what is expected of them, particularly in regard to courtesy and safety.

After the trip, the girls discuss and reflect on their trip. Follow-up activities may include dramatizations, stories, or art activities, such as paintings of what impressed them. They should send thank-you notes to anyone who helped make the trip possible or memorable, and they may include a painting or a poem they have written. They make plans for future trips, basing these plans on what they have learned, enjoyed, or need to practice.

Junior Girl Scouts

Junior Girl Scouts should read the sections in the *Junior Girl Scout Handbook* on planning trips and safety procedures.

With adult help, girls decide where they want to go. Girls plan the trip in patrols or small groups, keeping the trip's purpose in mind and including budgeting, pretrip skills, and tips for personal conduct and safety. Leaders advise girls as needed and help them keep their ideas realistic and fun for their age.

Badge activities suggest trips to all kinds of places in the community, as well as hikes, walks, and campouts. Junior Girl Scouts go on day trips in their own communities and to places of interest nearby. Eventually, their plans include longer trips, with stays in hotels or motels as well as camps.

Girl Scouts 11-14 years of age

Girl Scouts 11-14 years of age can go away for three days or longer if they have taken overnight trips. For example, they might go to a state capital or visit with groups in other parts of the country. Contacts with other groups provide ideas to start girls thinking.

Girl Scouts 11-14 years of age can combine camp living with exploration and travel, using a campsite as a base from which to take trips. Girls with specialized skills—such as horseback riding, biking, skiing, backpacking, or boating—may plan trips around those interests. Girls may also use these skills and interests to prepare for a national wider opportunity.

Leaders/advisors can encourage girls to share the excitement of their trip by making exhibits, showing slides, and illustrating log books for their families and friends and for community groups. After several trips, they can share their travel know-how with less experienced groups.

Girl Scouts 15 Years of Age and Older

Because Girl Scouts over 15 years of age usually have greater emotional, physical, and mental maturity than younger girls, they can benefit from more extensive travel. In addition, mature girls, experienced in travel or in planning, can work with less experienced girls or younger groups. They can help with the planning process, teach specific skills needed for a trip, or serve in a leadership role. They may also use the information in this chapter to prepare for a national or international wider opportunity.

Travel Procedures for Visiting the Juliette Gordon Low Girl Scout National Center

The Juliette Gordon Low Girl Scout National Center provides year-round educational program opportunities for traveling Junior, Cadette, and Senior Girl Scout groups. Reservations and council approval are required for visiting the Birthplace. Most programs are booked a minimum of one year in advance. Families and individuals do not need a reservation for a tour. The house is closed every Wednesday and some major holidays. For information about specific programs and days and hours of operation, or to request a copy of *Birthplace Bound*, a booklet summarizing educational programs, schedules, and fees as well as lodging, camping, restaurants, and sightseeing opportunities, contact the Center by calling (912) 233-4501, faxing (912) 233-4659, or writing the Juliette Low Center at 10 East Oglethorpe Avenue, Savannah, Georgia 31401.

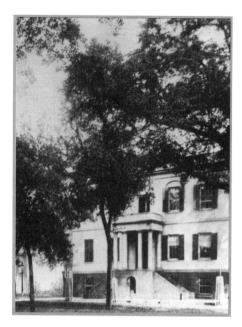

Travel Tips for All Trips

The trip must meet all appropriate Program Standards listed in chapter 6, "Girl Scout Program Standards." Pay particular attention to the appropriate girl/adult ratios for the different age levels.

The adults learn and share with the group ahead of time how to access the emergency medical system during trips. Emergency plans are made before departure.

Before a trip, all participants are briefed on:

◆ What to do if accidentally separated from the group

◆ What to do if emergency help is needed

◆ How to deal with the public in a tourist area

◆ How to perform basic first-aid procedures

◆ Expected behaviors

Find out in advance about the places to be visited:

◆ How long it will take to get there and the best means of transportation

◆ The availability of drinking water, restrooms, and eating places

◆ Visiting hours and the need, if any, for advance reservations

◆ Any physical barriers that cannot be accommodated

Allow enough time for eating, resting, and personal needs while traveling. Make alternative plans in case of bad weather or an emergency. When a large group plans to eat in a restaurant, make a reservation and, to save time, consider either ordering meals in advance or ordering the same menu for all. Arrive on time, or notify the restaurant if the group will be delayed. Ask about the inclusion of gratuities when a large group is served.

Be sure that each girl knows which adult or patrol leader she is responsible to while on the trip, and that each adult knows the names of the girls she is responsible for. Arrange for a back-home contact who will be available by phone during the trip. Inform that person of any delay or emergency along the way.

Use the buddy system when traveling. As part of trip preparation, discuss consideration for drivers and

other passengers. Wherever possible, arrange in advance for assigned seats in buses, trains, planes, or cars to ensure that all participants have seats. On longer trips, rotate seating periodically so that everyone gets a chance at the window seats. Remember to practice emergency evacuation procedures from vehicles.

When making reservations for overnight stops, find out whether there is a procedure for preregistering a large group. If there is, one person can check in for the entire group while the others remain in the bus or cars until accommodations are assigned.

It is not necessary to do everything as a group while traveling. Provisions can be made for breaking into smaller groups to pursue special interests and to have some unscheduled time to relax.

Checklist for Travel Readiness

Here is a checklist of general indicators for leaders and girls to look for to determine group readiness for a trip. Group consultants and others who review the travel plans should also find the checklist useful. Program services personnel can use the checklist as they approve travel plans, evaluate trips, and make trip recommendations.

The following statements show travel readiness:

1. The trip upholds Girl Scout policies and standards.

◆ The trip meets all appropriate Program Standards listed in chapter 6, "Girl Scout Program Standards."

2. There is communication with the council.

◆ All appropriate permissions have been obtained from the council.

◆ Leaders/advisors and girls know and follow council policies on camps and overnight trips, including procedures for handling emergencies.

◆ Council staff are informed of any changes in plans.

3. There is sound planning.

◆ The trip has a clear purpose, formulated and understood by the girls and adults.

◆ The trip is part of ongoing group activities, with all participants included in the planning steps.

◆ Girls work successfully in groups and accept the responsibilities involved in the trip.

◆ The proper number of adult chaperones who accept the responsibilities of the trip have been recruited.

◆ Girls and their parents or guardians support the project wholeheartedly; parents or guardians understand all plans and have confidence in the leadership.

- Girls and adults together make realistic, detailed plans well in advance.
- Plans consider the special abilities and the religious and ethnic diversity of the participants and of those they will interact with during the trip.
- Girls and adults learn in advance as much as possible about what they will be seeing and doing.
- The group seeks council guidance and approval on the best means of transportation for the trip.

4. Travel arrangements are made in advance.

- Time is provided for eating, sleeping, rest and relaxation, recreation, and personal needs.
- Mileage to be covered each day is reasonable for the terrain expected.
- Plans consider both drivers and passengers.
- Reservations for overnight accommodations are confirmed in writing, and all stopping places are planned in advance. Sufficient space is reserved so that each girl has her own bed.
- The entire itinerary is known to girls, adults, parents, the council, and the back-home emergency contact.

5. Business and money matters are

worked out.

- Girls and adults create a detailed, realistic budget, remembering to include such items as transportation, food, tips, insurance, recreation, admission fees, taxes, and emergency funds.
- Money-earning projects are carried on with the permission of the council and in accordance with Girl Scout policies and Program Standards.
- Personal and group expenses are defined. The amount of personal money needed and how those funds should be handled are determined in advance.
- Group travel funds are kept in a bank before the trip and carried in traveler's checks during the trip.
- One person is responsible for group funds and will keep a daily account of expenditures. However, all the cash and traveler's checks should not be held by just one person at any time during the trip.
- Decisions are made in advance about how to pay bills that occur before the trip, en route, and afterward.
- For overseas trips, most hospitals and doctors will require cash or credit card payments. Adults are ready to request hospital and doctors' bills in English to expedite

claims processing with the insurance company after returning home.

6. Members take responsibility for personal conduct and equipment.

- Girls and adults know what clothing and equipment to take and how to use and pack the equipment.
- When the group travels in uniform, all travelers have a Girl Scout uniform and wear it correctly. Girls and adults are encouraged to be in uniform at national centers and at other Girl Guide/Girl Scout activities or events.
- Girls understand their responsibilities as travelers. Everyone is briefed on appropriate conduct and safety precautions in public places, restrooms, escalators, and elevators, as well as on building stairs and the selected forms of transportation.
- Groups staying in hotels are prepared to take special precautions to protect their own safety and know what to do in case of fire. (See "Hotel Security and Safety Tips" on pages 146–147 in the appendix.)
- Girls and adults are prepared for new experiences and are open to appreciating local customs and foods. When traveling internationally, groups learn about local cus-

toms and behaviors in advance.

- Special equipment required, such as tents, bicycles, canoes, etc., is checked and ready well before the departure date.

- Individual limits on luggage and equipment are set and adhered to. Each person is able to carry her own individually identified belongings except when a special consideration, such as a disability, warrants alternative plans. All valuables are left at home.

7. Everyone knows and observes good health and safety practices.

- *Safety-Wise* is used when preparing for any trip. Girls and adults consult handbooks and leaders' guides for additional information.

- Required health examinations and immunizations are completed. Health records, medical waivers, necessary medications, eyeglass and contact lens prescriptions, and/or extra eyeglasses are taken along.

- Everyone is physically and mentally able to undertake the trip. Reasonable accommodations are made for girls who have disabilities.

- For trips of a day or more, at least one currently certified first-aider is present. The council office is contacted to determine the level of first-aid training needed. Provisions are made for first aid.

- For trips of three nights or more,

insurance coverage is obtained for the entire trip through the council under one of the optional accident or accident and sickness plans available. For international trips, request information from your council about the comprehensive foreign travel insurance and travel assistance program provided by Mutual of Omaha.

- Arrangements have been made for an adult contact back home for routine reporting as well as for emergencies.

- Written itineraries, including telephone numbers and addresses, are prepared for girls, their families, the council office, and the back-home contact. On overseas trips, the written itineraries include U.S. embassy and consulate locations.

- Everyone understands procedures for handling accidents, illnesses,

and emergencies.

- Trip leaders for specialized trips, such as canoeing or backpacking, have taken water safety and leadership training for the activity and are familiar with Girl Scout Program Standards and activity checkpoints set forth in *Safety-Wise.*

- Necessary insurance forms are carried, along with all important papers.

Tips for Girls Traveling Alone

The procedures for Cadette and Senior Girl Scouts traveling alone to and from a wider opportunity should help the girl feel comfortable and capable of traveling on her own and should include:

- Wider opportunity task group guidance through the application, acceptance, and trip-planning process.

- Assessment by the wider opportunity task group of the girl's maturity and ability to handle herself alone, including consultation with the girl's parents or guardian.

- Orientation on hotel security and safety. (See pages 146–147.)

- Provision of emergency forms, with names and telephone numbers of emergency contacts if the girl's family is not available;

arrangements for acceptance of emergency collect calls by emergency contacts. Note that the wider opportunity sponsor provides telephone numbers of emergency contacts at the event site or the arrival point.

◆ Advice to the girl and her family to book nonstop direct flights to and from the event whenever possible, and advice to have the travel agent alert the airline and airport personnel that the girl is traveling alone. Airlines provide extra help and support for minors traveling alone.

◆ When girls are traveling alone, in public places, it is not recommended that they wear name badges/tags that are visible to a casual passerby.

The council can provide the leader and the girl with additional information and advice to help ensure a safe trip.

Council-Sponsored Trips

Some councils arrange trips that are open to individual girls, such as camping, conferences, and volunteer service and leader-in-training projects. In sponsoring these trips, the council provides opportunities for girls to pursue special interests if they are willing to devote time to preparation.

Transportation and Travel

Transportation decisions are a very important part of trip planning. The first concern is always safety, but even with the greatest care, accidents can happen. Councils must understand safety requirements to evaluate and make recommendations on the kinds of transportation groups use and to determine what is best for a particular trip.

In planning a trip, leaders and girls must work closely with the council from the beginning. Girl Scout leaders are not authorized to sign agreements or contracts for renting or chartering vehicles, vessels, and aircraft. A written agreement is required even when there is no cost. All contracts and agreements must be submitted to the council to be signed by the person designated by the council board of directors.

Councils must have policies and procedures for transportation for group travel. Adults and girls must check with the council before proceeding to be sure they follow accepted practices. They must follow council guidelines to ensure that both they and the council are properly protected by liability insurance in the event of an accident. General liability and automobile liability policies cover claims or lawsuits arising out of an accident that occurs during a Girl Scout activity.

Auto Accident Facts and Safety Tips for Extended Trips

The following information and advice are great for any trip but are especially important on extended trips—to increase driving safety and awareness.

According to the National Safety Council, one motor vehicle death occurs every 12 minutes and one motor vehicle injury every 12 seconds. In the time it takes to go on a two-hour field trip with a group, there will be 10 motor vehicle deaths and 600 injuries across the country.

Over the last three years, almost 200 incidents have occurred to Girl Scouts in vehicles insured through the Girl Scout insurance program sponsored by Girl Scouts of the USA and Palmer & Cay. This means about 66 accidents each year, affecting close to one in three Girl Scout councils. Some were minor incidents, but unfortunately, others were much more serious. Serious injuries and deaths have occurred as a result of drivers falling asleep at the wheel, driving too fast and losing control of the vehicle, and making left turns into oncoming traffic.

Accidents do not always happen to the other person! Examples have just been given of accidents that happened to Girl Scouts. **Most of these accidents were preventable.** Everything a driver does to promote and increase safe driving practices will help prevent further personal tragedies.

THE TOP FIVE CAUSES OF AUTO ACCIDENTS ARE THE DRIVER:

- Not looking before backing up.
- Rear-ending another vehicle.
- Being distracted by passengers.
- Falling asleep at the wheel or driving while tired.
- Making a left turn into oncoming traffic.

Tips for Safety Talks with Drivers

While no one wants to be involved in an auto accident, there are auto accidents every day. Girl Scouts and their drivers have been involved in numerous auto accidents. Many of these accidents, which included serious injuries and deaths, were preventable. Drivers can avoid auto accidents by staying alert and using the following safe driving techniques:

- Not driving in bad weather, or if already on the road, slow down or pull as far off the road as possible and stop. Bad weather decreases visibility; wet roads reduce traction and cause skidding and increase the distance needed to stop.

- Always keeping the proper distance between your vehicles and the vehicles ahead. This allows time to respond. A three-second rule is useful. A driver watches the car ahead as it passes an object on the side of the road and counts "1000-1, 1000-2, 1000-3." If the driver passes that object before the end of the count, she or he is too close and needs to back off. If a van or a vehicle loaded with gear is being driven, the count should be increased to 1000-4. During bad weather, the driver increases

the count, as it will take longer to stop.

- Not driving while tired or taking medications that can induce drowsiness. You can actually "micro-sleep" while you drive, which is highly dangerous.

- Never taking your eyes off the road for any reason. To resolve an argument among the passengers, to read a map, or to use a cellular phone, pull off the road at an exit or rest area.

- Keeping your eyes on the road. Scan your mirrors frequently and watch the road on all sides. If there is a problem, you can stop or accurately determine how to avoid it. Also watch the brake lights of cars ahead and be alert for warning signs along the road.

- Driving with your headlights on and avoiding the blind spots of other vehicles, especially large trucks. Drivers use their turn signals when changing lanes or preparing to turn.

- Never speeding. Excessive speed can cause accidents because you need more time and distance to be able to react or stop.

- Wearing seat belts at all times. Require all passengers to buckle up before you start your vehicle.

Trip Planning Checklist

Use the following checklist when planning a trip:

- ☐ Review trip planning tips throughout *Safety-Wise*.
- ☐ Review your council's policies and procedures for trips.
- ☐ File trip plans according to your council's procedures.
- ☐ Check with your councils for insurance limits needed by drivers.
- ☐ Obtain insurance information from drivers.
- ☐ If renting vehicles, check with your council for procedures.
- ☐ Talk with all drivers about safe driving tips. In addition, discuss your expectations and the girls' expectations for the trip.
- ☐ Establish realistic schedules for the trips and safe places to stop for breaks along the way.
- ☐ Plan rest stops at least every two hours.
- ☐ Review council emergency procedures.
- ☐ Give important passenger information to each driver.
- ☐ Recruit an adequate number of adults to supervise girls and to relieve drivers on long trips.
- ☐ Discuss the trip thoroughly with the girls and agree on the ground rules.
- ☐ Establish that girls must not ride in the back of pickups or other trucks.
- ☐ Plan the route to the destination, obtain maps, and have toll money readily available, if needed.
- ☐ Prearrange meeting places for vehicles on the trip. There should be no driving in caravans or convoy formation.
- ☐ Plan to drive in daylight hours.
- ☐ Check cars for the number of factory-installed seat belts. There must be a seat belt for every rider.
- ☐ When using a cellular phone in an emergency, pull completely off the road and stop, set the emergency parking brake, and turn on flashers before dialing.
- ☐ Ask drivers to check all lights, signals, tires, windshield wipers, horns, and fluid levels before the trip.
- ☐ Plan to drive with the headlights on.
- ☐ Do not start a trip if bad weather will impair visibility and reduce safety.
- ☐ Place a first-aid kit in each vehicle.

Pledge Cards

The following pledge cards reinforce the idea that safety is the job of the driver and the passengers. Make copies and distribute them to drivers and Junior, Cadette, and Senior Girl Scouts who are passengers. All involved sign the cards to indicate that they have read them and understand the information. Further, signing signifies the driver's commitment to safe driving and the passenger's commitment to being a safe passenger.

SAFE PASSENGER PLEDGE

As a passenger on a Girl Scout trip, I understand it is my responsibility to help ensure our safety.
I pledge to:

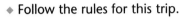

- Follow the rules for this trip.
- Keep my seat belt fastened around me.
- Practice good behavior—especially, to not yell, argue, or throw things.
- Ask whether there are any landmarks to find that would help the driver.
- Play games or music quietly with other passengers.

- Stay with my group when we stop.
- Alert the driver to any problems including a door being open, a missing buddy, a person or thing the driver can't see behind the vehicle as she or he is backing it up.
- Follow instructions given by the driver before and during the trip.

Passenger _____ **Date** _____

SAFE DRIVER PLEDGE

As a driver for a Girl Scout activity, I understand it is my responsibility to transport girls safely to
the scheduled activity and back to their parents or guardians. To ensure the safety of the girls,
I pledge to:

- Make sure that the vehicle is in safe operating condition before the trip.
- Ensure that everyone is wearing a seat belt any time the vehicle is moving.
- Drive within posted speed limits.
- Use turn signals for all turns and traffic lane changes.
- Yield to all oncoming traffic and be extra careful when making left turns.
- Keep at least a three-second interval between my vehicle and the vehicle in front of me when highway driving.

- Drive with extra caution during hours of darkness and any other time visibility is reduced or road conditions worsen.
- Plan extended trips to avoid driving in the dark.
- Never drive when sleepy.
- Take a rest break every two hours.
- Alternate drivers when I need a break.
- Drive no more than six hours a day.
- Never use a cellular phone while driving. I will pull over and stop, put the car in park, and put on flashing lights before dialing.

Driver _____ **Date** _____

GREAT TIPS FOR GREAT TRIPS!

- Be sure to have all important passenger information with you.
- Check that the vehicle is ready to go: wipers, tires, lights, signals, fluid levels, and horn.
- Put a first-aid kit, flashlight, and cellular phone on board.
- Know where you are going. Get directions and review a map if necessary.
- Ready to go? SEAT BELTS ON?
- Drive with your headlights on.
- Keep radio volume low enough to be able to hear other vehicles' horns.

- Always use your turn signals.
- Maintain proper distance from the cars ahead.
- Drive only at a safe, legal speed.
- Know what is around your vehicle. Check mirrors frequently. Look before backing up.
- Always yield the right of way!
- Stop and stretch every two hours.
- Slow down or pull off the road when weather makes road conditions worse.
- Always pull off the road and stop before using a cellular phone. Put car in park, turn on flashing lights, and then dial.

Have a great trip!

This information has been compiled by representatives of Girl Scout councils, Palmer & Cay, and the St. Paul Fire and Marine Insurance Company as members of a Participating Council Safety Group.

GREAT TIPS FOR GREAT TRIPS!

- Be sure to have all important passenger information with you.
- Check that the vehicle is ready to go: wipers, tires, lights, signals, fluid levels, and horn.
- Put a first-aid kit, flashlight, and cellular phone on board.
- Know where you are going. Get directions and review a map if necessary.
- Ready to go? SEAT BELTS ON?
- Drive with your headlights on.
- Keep radio volume low enough to be able to hear other vehicles' horns.

- Always use your turn signals.
- Maintain proper distance from the cars ahead.
- Drive only at a safe, legal speed.
- Know what is around your vehicle. Check mirrors frequently. Look before backing up.
- Always yield the right of way!
- Stop and stretch every two hours.
- Slow down or pull off the road when weather makes road conditions worse.
- Always pull off the road and stop before using a cellular phone. Put car in park, turn on flashing lights, and then dial.

Have a great trip, and deliver your precious cargo home safely!

This information has been compiled by representatives of Girl Scout councils, Palmer & Cay, and the St. Paul Fire and Marine Insurance Company as members of a Participating Council Safety Group.

Choosing Transportation

Before any mode of transportation is selected, make certain that the owner/operator is properly licensed and that the vehicle is registered, insured for liability, and well maintained. Check with your council for appropriate procedures.

Public Transportation

Transportation companies that commonly serve the public are called common carriers. These are trains and railroads, commercial airlines, bus lines, and ship lines and are usually preferable to charters, as they are subject to regulations that set standards for equipment, personnel, and insurance.

Any chartering of vehicles or watercraft needs the attention of appropriate legal counsel. This kind of activity should not be undertaken without council guidance.

Buses

To reach a location that is beyond scheduled routes, the group may want to charter a bus. Under the agreement, the bus company supplies the vehicle and the driver. The council must be involved in the selection and approval of bus companies.

Council volunteers and staff must check that vehicles have current registration, that state-mandated safety inspections have been passed, and that there are no obvious defects, such as bald tires, missing or broken lights, or cracked or broken glass (including mirrors and windshields). Contracts with vehicle owners should stipulate that it is the owner's responsibility to provide a vehicle in safe operating condition and to replace the vehicle or driver if problems develop.

All vehicles traveling on public roads should be equipped with first-aid kits, emergency lights/warning reflectors, and fire extinguishers. Whenever possible, vehicles should be equipped with communication devices such as radio phones or cellular phones. The phone numbers for appropriate contacts should be readily available.

The council should have a current certificate of insurance from the bus company on file. When buses are leased or rented with the bus company's insurance, the council should check with its own insurance agent to determine the minimum amount of insurance that is required by local or state statute.

When chartering, renting, or borrowing any bus, the council checks for the following and requests verified documentation, as appropriate:

- Liability and collision/comprehensive insurance for the vehicle
- Workers' compensation insurance for the driver
- Qualifications, training, and licensing of the driver
- Relief-driver availability
- Familiarity of driver with vehicle
- Sufficient seating and luggage space
- Appropriate emergency equipment

Most states require a vehicle to have a specified minimum amount of liability insurance. However, some states require none, and the council must judge whether the state minimum is reasonable for the Girl Scout event. It must also be aware of requirements in other states through which the vehicle will pass. The leader must contact the council to find out the amount of liability insurance needed.

Most charter agreements include the provision of a driver.

Some insurance carriers provide insurance only when the owner/operator is using the bus for the owner's purposes—for example, when the school district is using the bus for school district activities. The council needs to verify that the bus's insurance will be valid when the bus is used for Girl Scout purposes, whether or not the Girl Scouts pay to use the bus.

The council gives the group a list of transportation providers that it can use when planning Girl Scout activities. Councils should use local or state regulatory authorities to help in determining reputable transportation providers.

Private Passenger Vehicles

Cars, vans, and station wagons are all suitable for transportation—provided each passenger has a proper seat and seat belt, the vehicle is not overcrowded, there is adequate insurance, and the vehicle is well maintained. Girls under 12 years of age should sit in the back seat whenever possible to reduce the possibility of injury during the deployment of an airbag in the front passenger seat. The front seat should be pushed back as far as possible to reduce the potential for injury to front-seat occupants. All riders must have their seat belts buckled whenever the vehicle is in motion.

All states regulate drivers' licensing and vehicle registration. Most states dictate the minimum amount of liability insurance required. The leader should ask the council how much liability insurance is required for the event/activity being planned. In the event of an accident, the owner's vehicle insurance is the primary applicable insurance.

Leased or Rented Vehicles

Read all rental agreements carefully to comply with their terms and avoid surprises. Note especially the type and the amount of insurance carried by the rental agency. Rental agreements often specify the minimum age of the driver, from 21 to 25.

Know who is responsible for damage to or loss of the vehicle itself. State laws vary greatly on what rental agencies can sell to and/or require of renters. Check with the council to ensure that its non-owned automobile coverage will be effective if needed.

Special Vehicles

Commercial vehicles without seats, such as flatbed or panel trucks, must never be used to carry passengers. These are utility vehicles designed to transport property. Vehicles such as reconditioned buses that are handmade or that cannot be registered as vehicles should not be used to transport passengers. Only vehicles designed to carry passengers can be used to transport Girl Scouts. Drivers of vehicles that hold more than 15 passengers must have a commercial driver's license.

Recreational vehicles. When using these vehicles, such as snowmobiles, note the following:

- The owners should have appropriate liability insurance.
- The vehicles must be maintained in accordance with the manufacturer's specifications.
- The vehicles should be driven by experienced operators over tracks that are free of such obstacles as rocks, fences, barbed wire, and low-hanging branches.

- The vehicles must be registered and/or inspected in compliance with the law.

Campers. Passengers must be transported in seats designed by the manufacturer for sitting and seat belts must be worn. Transporting people any other way may void insurance coverage. Cargo must be safely stowed so that sudden stops or impact will be unlikely to hurt passengers. People should not be transported in five-wheel camper/trailers, in campers that fit onto pickup flatbeds, or in any trailer body without direct access to the driver.

Air Transportation

Regularly scheduled airlines are recommended for Girl Scout group travel. These air carriers provide many choices, with varying costs. Before making a decision, discuss with a travel agent the differences in cost based on advance booking and off-season and group fares.

Charter flights by Girl Scout groups involve legal and financial responsibilities, and the purchase of additional, special liability insurance. The council must approve and sign any agreements to charter flights. Generally, chartering planes is not recommended, as it is impractical for Girl Scout councils.

Watercraft Transportation

In recent years, both federal and state regulation of boating have been increasing. The council must be sure that craft used meet the standards of the regulatory agency in the jurisdiction. Chartering boats longer than 16 feet, with or without a crew, is not recommended. Special licenses for certain crew members are usually required, and Admiralty Law usually makes the charterer responsible not only for any damage to the boat, but also for damage to other boats and pollution of waterways, and may even require removal of sunken vessels from navigable waters.

All vessels carrying passengers must be registered or documented according to federal regulations and state statute. They are also inspected according to U.S. Coast Guard or state regulation (depending on number of passengers, size of vessel, means of propulsion, and water routes). Vessel operators are licensed as required by federal regulations or state statute.

PFDs (life jackets) are available in an appropriate size for each passenger and are easily accessible. Vessels are not overloaded. The number of persons aboard must not exceed the recommended or certified capacity. Luggage and equipment are stowed securely and balanced to help keep the vessel stable.

The securing of adequate liability insurance for chartered passenger-carrying vessels should be thoroughly investigated before entering any charter arrangements.

Trips to Other Countries

As noted on page 46, girls who take overnight trips may eventually progress to trips outside the country. Trips to Canada or Mexico introduce girls to international travel and allow them to practice being good ambassadors. Trips abroad require two or three years of preparation and relatively few Girl Scout groups or council-sponsored groups undertake them.

Before initiating a trip to another country, girls and leaders should have demonstrated to the council their ability to plan, organize, budget, accept responsibility, observe emergency and safety measures, work together as a group, and evaluate their experiences through a variety of successful short and extended trips.

When there is interest in traveling outside the country, leaders and girls should inform the council and get permission to plan the trip. They should work with the council from the beginning and establish a timetable and checkpoints for reporting progress as plans develop. They should secure final council permission and other permissions as required along the way.

Preparation Packet

Girl Scout groups planning an international trip can obtain a preparation packet from the council. This packet contains advice on immunizations and other health precautions, working with a travel agent, obtaining passports and other needed documents, learning about other countries and cultures, financing an international trip, what to take and how to pack, resources on Girl Scouting and Girl Guiding around the world, and making your travel dreams come true. Also included are helpful hints from girls who have traveled abroad. All Girl Scout groups planning trips to other countries are advised to obtain this packet.

Do not contact Girl Guide/Girl Scout association offices in other countries when planning a trip. Most Girl Guide/Girl Scout offices are very small, with only a handful of employees. To avoid overwhelming these people with correspondence, international commissioners carry on all communication between Girl Guide/Girl Scout organizations. Write to GSUSA's international commissioner at: International Commissioner, c/o International Relations, GSUSA, 420 Fifth Avenue, New York, N.Y. 10018-2798.

Travel Procedures for Visiting WAGGGS Centers or Member Countries

Groups wishing to stay at a world center or a Girl Guide hostel or wishing to visit the Girl Guide/Girl Scout headquarters in countries where there is a WAGGGS organization must follow specific procedures.

Procedures for travel to Canada, along with an application form, can be found in the appendix. (See pages 141–142.) Councils may reproduce the procedures and form as needed.

Intent to Travel Forms A and B are also in the appendix (pages 144–145), along with procedures for their use (page 143), and may be reproduced by councils as needed.

◆ Intent to Travel Form A is for travelers who plan to stay at a world center or Girl Guide hostel.

◆ Intent to Travel Form B is for individuals or groups who plan to visit a world center or a member country of the World Association of Girl Guides and Girl Scouts while traveling abroad and wish to obtain a Card of Introduction.

All Girl Guide and Girl Scout associations recognize the Card of Introduction as the standard form of introduction. Through GSUSA's membership in the World Association, the card is available to Girl Scouts to facilitate contact with Girl Guides in the countries to be visited. However, the card does not entitle travelers to request hospitality or services. Such requests are inappropriate and should not be made.

Timetable

One to two years before the trip, the leader planning to visit or stay at a world center or Girl Guide hostel completes Intent to Travel Form A and sends it to the council. The council sends a copy to GSUSA's Membership and Program Services, provides guidance for the group, and reminds the leader to confirm dates, itinerary, insurance coverage, and the list of travelers (girls and adults) six to eight weeks before departure. Membership and Program Services responds to the leader, sending the information requested on the Intent to Travel Form.

Six to eight weeks before the trip, the leader confirms with the council the dates, itinerary, insurance coverage, and list of travelers. The council sends the endorsed Intent to Travel Form B to Membership and Program Services at GSUSA. Cards of Introduction are sent to the leader. Travelers requesting Cards of Introduction less than a month in advance cannot be assured of receiving them before departure.

Individuals may follow the same procedures, notifying the council of travel plans in advance if planning to visit or stay at a world center. Or if they need only Cards of Introduction, individual travelers may inform the council six to eight weeks in advance of their plans, travel dates, itinerary, and names of travelers. The council sends an endorsed copy of Intent to Travel Form B to Membership and Program Services. A Card of Introduction is sent to the individual.

After Any Trip

After any trip, all bills should be paid promptly. Girls and adults should write thank-you letters to people who helped along the way and return borrowed or rented equipment in good condition.

Evaluate the trip with the girls. Discuss what was fun and worthwhile, decide what the group would like to change or eliminate on future trips, and report back to the council with the group's evaluation.

Build new activities based on the group's travel experiences. Share the experiences with others, and don't forget the people in the community who helped with the group's preparations. Have the group pass tips along to other Girl Scouts planning similar trips. Encourage girls to keep in touch with friends made along the way. Someday these friends may visit your area.

PART

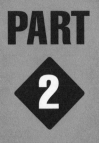

Girl Scout Program Standards and Activity Checkpoints

Girl Scout Program Standards

The Girl Scout program is an informal educational program designed to help girls put into practice the fundamental principles of the Girl Scout Movement as set forth in the Preamble. It is carried out in small groups with adult leadership and provides a wide range of activities developed around the interests and needs of girls.

—Constitution of Girl Scouts of the United States of America, Article III

The 35 Program Standards describe the basic philosophy of the Girl Scout program and the basic levels of health and safety that must be provided to girls. Every Girl Scout adult who is involved with girls, either directly or indirectly, must be familiar with these standards. Each Program Standard specifies the elements of a quality program experience for girls. As a whole, they ensure that all Girl Scouts will benefit from a rewarding educational experience carried out in a way that safeguards the health, safety, and general well-being of all participants.

Each standard is followed by a set of statements that further describe the standard, and provide examples and details to more fully illustrate what is done in order to meet the standard.

The standards are organized into five major sets: Girl Scout Program, Adult Leadership Roles and Responsibilities, Group Management, Transportation, and Money Earning/Group Financing.

Some standards require greater explanation than others, but this does not mean that any standard is more important than another. When the information in one standard draws upon important information found in other standards, those standards are listed in the information below the standard. Sometimes you may be referred to another section of the book. These directions are important to follow, since they will provide you with critical information related to the standard. You will also find references to other Girl Scout resources that contain more information related to the standard.

Girl Scout Program

STANDARD 1

Girl Scout Program—Its Foundation and Goals

Program experiences and activities meet the needs and interests of girls, are based on the Girl Scout Promise and Law, and enable girls to grow and develop, as described in the four Girl Scout Program Goals.

The Girl Scout program has four fundamental goals, and the experiences and activities enable each girl to:

Develop to her full individual potential.

- Foster feelings of self-acceptance and unique self-worth.
- Promote her perception as competent, responsible, and open to new experiences and challenges.
- Offer opportunities to learn new skills.
- Encourage personal growth.
- Allow her to utilize and practice her talents and abilities.

To relate to others with increasing understanding, skill, and respect.

- Help each girl develop sensitivity to others and respect for their needs, feelings, and rights.

- Promote an understanding and appreciation of individual, cultural, religious, and racial differences.
- Foster the ability to build friendships and working relationships.

Develop values to guide her actions and to provide the foundation for sound decision-making.

- Help her develop a meaningful set of values and ethics that will guide her actions.
- Foster an ability to make decisions that are consistent with her values and that reflect respect for the rights and needs of others.
- Empower her to act upon her values and convictions.
- Encourage her to reexamine her ideals as she matures.

To contribute to the improvement of society through the use of her abilities and leadership skills, working in cooperation with others.

- Help her develop concern for the well-being of her community and its people.
- Promote an understanding of how the quality of community life affects her own life and the whole of society.
- Encourage her to use her skills to work with others for the benefit of all.

The four Program Goals provide direction for Girl Scout program that is adapted to meet the developmental, educational, emotional, and social needs and interests of girls at five age levels.

The age levels are:
- Daisy Girl Scouts
  (K–grade 1 or 5–6 years old)
- Brownie Girl Scouts
  (grades 1–3 or 6-8 years old)
- Junior Girl Scouts
  (grades 3–6 or 8–11 years old)
- Girl Scouts
  (grades 6–9 or 11–14 years old)
- Girl Scouts
  (grades 9–12 or 14–17 years old)

Girls with mental retardation should be registered as closely as possible to their chronological age. They wear the uniform of that age level. Make any required adaptations to the ongoing activities of the age level to which the group belongs. Young women who are mentally retarded may retain their girl membership through their 21st year and then move into an adult membership category.

Program age level is determined by the current membership year beginning October 1st.

STANDARD 2

General Activities

Program activities include a balance of subject and interest areas. The types of activities are determined in partnership by the girls and their leaders and reflect the girls' needs and interests, physical and emotional readiness, skill level, and preparation. The activities provide for progressive learning experiences, both at the current age level and in preparation for the next one.

Activities include opportunities for:

◆ Cooperative learning experiences
◆ Experiential learning
◆ Individual and group participation
◆ Development of values
◆ Decision-making
◆ Skill building
◆ Exploration of roles and contributions of women past, present, and future
◆ Respect for and understanding and appreciation of cultural, religious, ethnic, and racial diversity

Vary activities in type and subject matter.

Plan activities with sensitivity to varying needs and abilities of girls in language skills, proficiency in English, and mental and physical disabilities.

Use the handbooks, awards books, and other supplemental resources to plan and guide the activities.

For additional guidance on specific activities, see chapter 7, "Activity Checkpoints."

Ceremonies are held to emphasize important moments in Girl Scouting, including:

◆ Investiture
◆ Rededication
◆ Court of Awards
◆ Fly-Up and Bridging
◆ Thinking Day
◆ Girl Scouts' Own

(*Ceremonies in Girl Scouting* and the various handbooks provide further information on these and other ceremonies.)

STANDARD 3

Health, Safety, and Security— Activity Planning and Implementation

At all times, the health, safety, and security of girls are paramount. All activities are planned and carried out so as to safeguard the health, safety, and general well-being of girls and adults. Girls and adults follow proper safety practices at all times.

In planning an activity with the group, the leader should note the abilities of each girl and carefully consider the progression of skills required to go from the easiest part of the activity to the most difficult. She should make sure that the complexity of the activity does not exceed the girls' individual skill levels, bearing in mind that skill levels will decline when the participants are tired, hungry, or under stress.

Girls and leaders/advisors should learn and follow health and safety practices as outlined in this text and in each of the basic Girl Scout program resources.

To avoid needless risks in any group, maintain an effective level of disci-

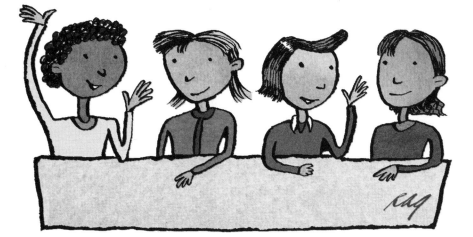

pline.

Before a girl participates in physically demanding activities, obtain a health history (see glossary) and an activity permission form (see page 137) signed by the parent or guardian. Information in a health history is confidential.

Before a girl participates in resident camping, in a trip of more than three nights, or in contact sports on an organized competitive basis, a record of health examination (see glossary) given by a licensed physician, nurse practitioner, physician's assistant or registered nurse within the preceding 24 months is required. See page 39.

If there is a religious reason for not having such an examination, obtain a signed statement by the religious leader to that effect. Ask your council for an appropriate form, if necessary.

Anyone who has a known complicating medical problem, or who has had a serious illness or injury or an operation since her last health examination, submits a written statement from her health care provider or religious authority, if her religion precludes the use of a physician, giving permission to participate in any activity that normally requires a current health history or health examination.

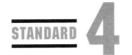

STANDARD 4

International

Girl Scouting is part of a worldwide movement, and program activities emphasize this international dimension.

Girls learn the significance of the World Pin and the meaning of the World Association of Girl Guides and Girl Scouts (WAGGGS).

Program activities for girls promote multicultural understanding and appreciation of diversity—geographic, economic, racial, ethnic, religious, etc.

Girls are familiar with the activities in their handbooks and other program resources containing Try-Its, badge activities, and interest projects that inform them about the international scope of the Girl Scout/Girl Guide movement.

Girls learn about their responsibilities and potential to contribute to a global society.

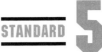

STANDARD 5

Service

Service is inherent in the Girl Scout Promise and Law and is given without expectation of payment or reward. All girls take part in service activities or projects.

The girls and the needs of the community determine service activities or projects.

Councils provide support to girls in identifying potential service projects, locating resources, and planning service projects.

Awards are not provided for hours of service. However, girls may be recognized for special training, skill development, leadership, and accomplishments, and some form of written documentation indicating the service rendered may be given to girls for their records.

STANDARD 6

Experiences Beyond the Group

Girls have experiences that broaden their perspectives and enable them to interact with individuals beyond their immediate group. Program activities provide girls with opportunities to have experiences beyond regular group meetings.

Inform parents or guardians and get written consent when activities take place outside the scheduled meeting place. See Standard 10.

Girls should have the opportunity to interact with other groups at the same and at different age levels.

Refer to chapter 5, "Planning Trips with Girl Scouts," for further information.

STANDARD 7

Outdoor Education

Activities carried out in outdoor settings are an important part of Girl Scout program for each age level. The leader receives the appropriate training from her council to help her guide preparation for and implementation of outdoor activities.

All activities in an outdoor setting reflect an understanding of the importance of conserving and caring for the environment and protecting wildlife.

Prior to their activities, girls learn about and practice skills they will use.

Outdoor Education in Girl Scouting provides information and guidance for outdoor-related activities.

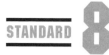

STANDARD 8

Girl Scout Camping

Girl Scout camping provides girls with a fun and educational group living experience that links Girl Scout program with the natural surroundings and contributes to each camper's mental, physical, social, and spiritual growth.

Leaders/advisors receive council training specifically designed to increase their skills in planning and managing the group camping experience before taking girls group camping.

Girls and their leaders/advisors work with the Girl Scout council in planning a Girl Scout camping experience. See Program Standards 6, 13, 14, 18, 22, 23, 24, 25, 26 and the activity checkpoints for Group Camping (pages 87–88).

Girls and adults prepare for the camping experience by learning basic outdoor skills and practicing minimal-impact camping skills.

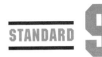

STANDARD 9

Girl Scout Awards

Girl Scout awards acknowledge a girl's accomplishments and attainment of specified requirements. Leaders work in partnership with girls to decide when awards such as Try-Its, badges, pins, or patches have been completed. At all times, adults play a key role in stressing the quality of the program experience over quantity of awards.

A leader/advisor should help girls understand the purpose of doing the activities for each award.

Girls choose the awards they will work on. A leader can guide a girl in choosing awards that suit her specific interests, talents, and abilities.

Girls may sometimes get too focused on the quantity of awards earned rather than the quality of the learning experience. Program activities are not designed only to fulfill award requirements. A leader should help girls appreciate the fun and value of doing something for its own sake, not just to obtain an award.

Girls may need help in planning the steps and activities needed to complete an award.

Credit is given for continuity of membership and for badges and activities, when properly recorded, to girls who have been affiliated with other Girl Scout groups or with recognized organizations within WAGGGS.

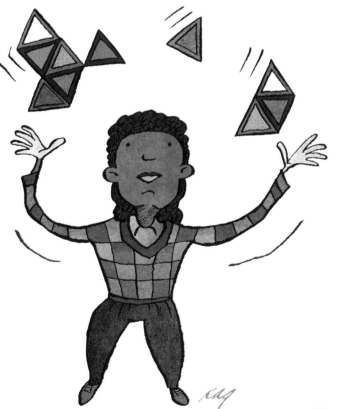

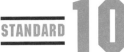

STANDARD 10

Parental Permission

Written permission from a parent or legal guardian is obtained for participation in Girl Scouting. Leaders and girls are responsible for informing parents or guardians of the purpose of Girl Scouting; of the date, time, and place of meetings; and of the type of activities included in group plans. When activities take place outside of the scheduled meeting place, involve overnight travel, or focus on sensitive or controversial topics, parents and guardians are informed and asked to provide additional written consent.

A leader/advisor must consult with her council representatives before doing overnight trips or any activities beyond those in this publication, or activities on sensitive or controversial issues. See page 40 for further information.

Before a leader/advisor develops plans for these activities, she must inform parents and guardians and discuss these activities with them. Girl members, regardless of age, are required to have written parent/guardian permission when required by the council.

Next, a leader/advisor gets a parent's or guardian's written permission for every girl wishing to participate in an activity, or a series of activities that is held at a different place and time from the regularly scheduled meeting place and time, or that involves unusual risks or controversial issues.

A leader/advisor can ask for her council's assistance concerning communication with a parent or guardian whose language she doesn't speak. The leader can request council assistance in helping a parent or guardian to overcome barriers to participation and input to group activities.

A leader/advisor should use parent permission forms provided by the council or get her council's input in developing permission forms for special activities.

Girl Scout Membership Pins and Uniforms

All Girl Scout members wear the Membership Pin when participating in Girl Scout activities. Since Girl Scouting is a uniformed organization, girl and adult members are informed, at the time they become members, that they are entitled to wear the Girl Scout uniform appropriate for their age level. Although the wearing of the uniform is encouraged, it should be clearly conveyed that the wearing of the uniform is not required to be a Girl Scout.

Members who do not own uniforms wear the Girl Scout Membership Pin appropriate for their age level.

Uniforms are not required for members to participate in Girl Scout activities.

Girl Scout uniforms can be an important contributor to group identity and promote a greater sense of unity and parity among members at each age level.

Guidelines for wearing the uniform appropriately are followed. The handbooks, leaders' guides, and GSUSA's Web site (www.girlscouts.org/girls) contain specific details.

When appropriate, the official uniform is used to identify traveling groups or individuals representing the organization.

 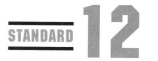

Girl/Adult Partnership

Girls and their leaders work as partners in planning and decision-making. Tasks are assigned with sensitivity to girls' developmental maturity and are commensurate with their abilities. Each girl is encouraged to proceed at her own pace. With each age level, the girls' opportunities to act independently and handle responsibilities increase.

To develop leadership skills, girls use simple forms of government, as outlined in the girls' handbooks.

The amount of guidance needed by the girls is matched to their age and maturity. Daisy Girl Scouts depend largely on their leader's/advisor's direction, while Girl Scouts 11 years of age and older plan with maximum independence. See pages 23–24.

Leaders/advisors can receive support from their Girl Scout council in addressing special needs of girls in the group. Refer to *Focus on Ability* for additional information on working with girls with disabilities.

A leader/advisor, program consultant, or outside instructor working with girls needs to have the skills, competencies, and preparation required for the type of activity she or he is conducting and the activity's level of difficulty.

Leaders/advisors assist girls in:

- Learning decision-making skills
- Assuming a variety of responsibilities
- Selecting activities that match abilities and encourage growth
- Proceeding at their own pace
- Recognizing that learning experiences involve both success and failure

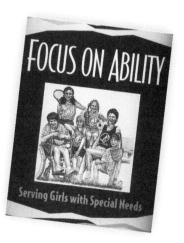

Adult Leadership Roles and Responsibilities

STANDARD 13

Leadership of Groups

Each group has at least one adult leader and one or more assistant leaders. Because the female role model is essential to fulfilling the purpose of Girl Scouting, at least one member of the leadership team must be an adult female.

The adult leaders/advisors must be at least 18 years of age or at the age of majority defined by the state if it is older than 18. Leaders/advisors are trained as specified by the council. In addition, an active group committee of registered adult members provides ongoing support to the group.

During all group meetings and related small-group activities, the leader/advisor, assistant leader, or other responsible adult designated by the leader or by the council is present, and at least one of these must be an adult female not related to the other adults.

There may be trips when fathers or male leaders/advisors are part of the group. It is not appropriate for males to sleep in the same space with girl members. They may participate only if separate sleeping quarters and bathrooms are available for their use. In some circumstances, such as a museum or mall overnight with hun-

dreds of girls, this type of accommodation may not be possible. If this is the case, men should not be part of the adults supervising girls in the sleeping area at the event. The adult-to-girl ratio for the trip will need to be adjusted accordingly.

Recommended ratios of adults to girls are:

- For meetings, two adults to every:
  - 10 Daisy Girl Scouts
  - 20 Brownie Girl Scouts
  - 25 Junior Girl Scouts
  - 25 Girl Scouts 11 to 14 years of age
  - 30 Girl Scouts 15 years of age or older

Plus one adult to each additional:
  - 5 Daisy Girl Scouts
  - 8 Brownie Girl Scouts
  - 10 Junior Girl Scouts
  - 12 Girl Scouts 11 to 14 years of age
  - 15 Girl Scouts 15 years of age or older

- For events, trips, and group camping, two adults to every:
  - 5 Daisy Girl Scouts*
  - 12 Brownie Girl Scouts
  - 16 Junior Girl Scouts
  - 20 Girl Scouts 11 to 14 years of age
  - 24 Girl Scouts 15 years of age or older

Plus one adult to each additional:
  - 3 Daisy Girl Scouts*
  - 6 Brownie Girl Scouts

8 Junior Girl Scouts

10 Girl Scouts 11 to 14 years of age

12 Girl Scouts 15 years of age or older

The group leadership team helps to recruit three to six members for the group committee and keeps them informed about the group plans. The group committee members are registered Girl Scout adults who provide the principal support to the leader/advisor by supplying transportation, assistance with projects, child care support, leader/advisor substitutes, etc.

A member of the group's sponsoring group is on the group committee. The committee is the communications link between the sponsor and the group.

Senior Girl Scouts who are Leaders-in-Training (LIT) and Counselors-in-Training (CIT) may supplement the regular adult leadership requirements but cannot substitute for adults.

Any adult volunteer whose behavior is not in keeping with the standards set forth in this book as well as those established by the council may be asked to relinquish her or his position.

* Under the leadership of the group leader, and with parents, guardians, or other family members participating, a Daisy Girl Scout group may participate in an occasional overnight camping experience.

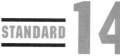

STANDARD 14

Health, Safety, and Security— Adult Supervision and Preparation

Proper adult supervision and guidance for each activity are essential. Adults with requisite expertise are part of the adult leadership when implementing activities. Adequate training and preparation for girls and adults precede participation in any activity.

Before doing any activity, review the general health and safety considerations. (See pages 78–83.)

Chapter 7, "Activity Checkpoints," provides specific information. When an activity being considered is not listed, contact a council representative, program consultant, adviser, and/or qualified personnel to provide direction and guidance, and to grant approval as required. Check page 80 to determine if the activity is not permitted as a Girl Scout program activity.

When an activity is planned on a topic of a sensitive or controversial nature, parents and the council are informed and permission is received before proceeding. (See Standard 10.)

When any activity is planned in which special equipment, training, or expertise is required, consult the council to ensure proper approval, supervision, and insurance coverage. See page 79 for instructions.

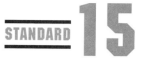

STANDARD 15

Council Support to Adult Leadership

All adults within the Girl Scout council work in concert to ensure the highest quality program experience for girls. Communication and cooperation are essential for providing training, giving ongoing support to groups, and obtaining appropriate activity approvals.

Group leaders/advisors and assistant leaders take advantage of basic and advanced program training and other adult education opportunities provided by the council or by council-approved outside organizations.

The leader/advisor obtains council permission for money-earning projects, overnight trips, and sensitive issues discussions, and keeps the council informed of ongoing group activities. Refer to the chapter "Planning Trips with Girl Scouts" on pages 44–60 for detailed guidance.

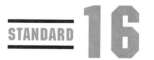

STANDARD 16

Program Consultants

The regular adult leadership of any Girl Scout group is complemented by program consultants who possess technical competence and the ability to share specialized skills.

See pages 17 and 139.

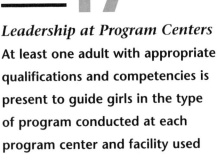

STANDARD 17

Leadership at Program Centers

At least one adult with appropriate qualifications and competencies is present to guide girls in the type of program conducted at each program center and facility used for Girl Scout program activities. Additional adults trained for their particular roles are present in numbers required to provide adequate adult guidance for the ages of the girls, the size of the group, and the nature of the activity.

The average ratios of girls to adults in a program center are two adults (**at least one of whom is female**) to every:

10 Daisy Girl Scouts

20 Brownie Girl Scouts

25 Junior Girl Scouts

25 Girl Scouts 11 to 14 years of age

30 Girl Scouts 15 years of age or older

Plus one adult for each additional:

5 Daisy Girl Scouts

8 Brownie Girl Scouts

10 Junior Girl Scouts

12 Girl Scouts 11to 14 years of age

15 Girl Scouts 15 years of age or older

Centers and facilities operated by a Girl Scout council meet the guidelines in *Safety Management at Girl Scout Sites and Facilities* and are accessible to girls with disabilities.

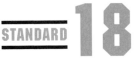

STANDARD 18

Adult Leadership—Girl Scout Camps

All Girl Scout camps are staffed by adults who possess the qualifications and necessary competencies for the positions held.

Each group will be led by adults, at least one of whom is an adult female.

See Standards 14, 15, and 22.

Camps operated by the Girl Scout council meet the guidelines in *Safety Management at Girl Scout Sites* and Facilities and are accessible to girls with disabilities.

Group Management

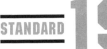

STANDARD 19

Pluralism and Diversity of Groups

Girl Scout groups reflect the diversity of the community. All girls are welcome regardless of socioeconomic status; racial, ethnic, cultural, or religious background; or disability.

Leaders and girls show respect for the beliefs and practices of all religious, ethnic, racial, linguistic, and socioeconomic sectors, as well as the varying levels of physical and mental ability in the group membership.

In choosing meeting places, selecting meeting dates and times, planning activities, considering schedules for trips, making group menus, etc., a leader considers the needs, resources, safety and security practices, and beliefs of all members, and the special needs of any members who have disabilities. See the appendix, page 140, for information on choosing appropriate sites.

The group committee and program consultants should reflect the diversity of the community.

See Standard 1 for guidelines related to serving girls with mental retardation. Refer to *Focus on Ability* for guidance on working with girls who have special needs.

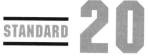

STANDARD 20

Size of Groups

Girls participate in groupings large enough to provide experience in self-government and small enough to allow for the development of the individual girl.

Ratios of girls to adults provide appropriate adult leadership. (See the guidelines for Program Standard 13.)

It is recommended that the group sizes be as follows:

Daisy Girl Scouts   5–15 girls
Brownie Girl Scouts   10–25 girls
Junior Girl Scouts   10–30 girls
Girl Scouts 11 to 14
    years of age   5–30 girls
Girl Scouts 15 years of
    age or older   5–30 girls

A group consists of at least five girls from more than one family.

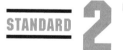

STANDARD 21

Meeting and Activity Planning

Groups meet often enough to fulfill the needs and interests of girls and to maintain continuity of their program experience.

The schedule of meetings and other activities is worked out by the girls in partnership with the leaders or other adults who work with them.

When planning meeting times, con-sider school schedules, family needs, scheduled events, religious holidays, safety concerns, and availability of transportation and meeting places to ensure full participation.

STANDARD 22

Meeting Places/Camps/Sites

All meeting places, camps, and other sites used for Girl Scout program activities provide a safe, clean, and secure environment and allow for participation of all girls.

Make sure that all places selected for activities are easily accessible to all members, including girls with disabilities.

The meeting area meets the following criteria:

- It is safe, secure, clean, properly ventilated, heated, lit, free from hazards, and has at least two exits.
- The area is large enough for a variety of activities.
- First-aid equipment is on hand.
- It has accessible toilets and sanitary facilities, including facilities designed to accommodate those with disabilities.
- It is accessible by telephone or other communication equipment.
- Emergency exits are functioning, easily accessible, adequate, and well marked.
- Adequate lighting is present.
- All pets are restrained away from the meeting area while girls are present.

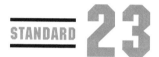

STANDARD 23

Girl Scout Camps

All Girl Scout camps are operated in compliance with Girl Scout guidelines and local and state laws for maximum protection of campers' health, safety, and security, and with regard to protection of the natural environment.

Girls are trained in outdoor living skills, health and safety procedures, and minimal impact camping.

Camps operated by a Girl Scout council meet the guidelines in *Safety Management at Girl Scout Sites and Facilities.*

Follow council procedures when making arrangements for girls to attend Girl Scout camp.

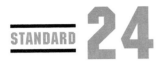

STANDARD 24

Overnight Trips, Camping

All sites and facilities used for overnight trips or camping are approved by the Girl Scout council.

The leader must inform the council of any planned overnight trips and obtain needed permission. See Standards 3, 6, 8, 13, 14, and 15.

Transportation

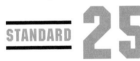

STANDARD 25

Private Transportation

Private passenger cars and vans may be used during Girl Scout activities. They must be properly registered, insured, and operated by adults with a valid license for the type and size of vehicle used. Any other form of private transportation may be used only after council approval has been obtained.

The number of passengers in the vehicle does not exceed the intended passenger limits. Each person has her or his own seat and is buckled into a seat belt.

Provide enough space for luggage and equipment and stow it securely.

Vehicles are used for their intended purpose. Trucks and similar vehicles used to transport equipment and supplies are not used to transport anyone in the area designed for cargo. Trailers or other towed vehicles are not used to transport passengers. Exception: Vehicles designed for hauling and in good condition may be used for hayrides on private property or for floats in parades. (For further information, see pages 131–133.)

Vehicles designed primarily to serve as recreational homes are used to transport only the number of persons for which there are specifically designed passenger seats and seat belts.

All vehicles are equipped with a first-aid kit and any federal- or state-required safety equipment (for example, spare tire, reflective devices, fire extinguishers).

The section on transportation on pages 57–59 should be consulted for further information about arranging transportation. See auto safety tips on pages 52–56.

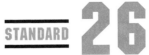

STANDARD 26

Public Transportation

Public transportation and regularly scheduled airlines, buses, trains, and vessels are used whenever possible.

See Program Standard 25 and pages 57–59.

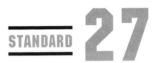

STANDARD 27

Travel Procedures

All travel procedures and preparations provide adequate adult supervision and maximum safety.

Follow your local Girl Scout council's group transportation procedures.

Train all girls and review all safety rules and procedures before the trip. All passengers are considerate of the driver and observe all safe conduct rules for the form of transportation used. (See pages 52–56.)

Provide adequate adult supervision. (See Program Standard 13.) Adults use procedures such as counting heads or buddies at each stop to ensure that everyone is accounted for.

Leave a trip plan with a designated person in the council.

In planning any trip, follow all recommendations in chapter 5, "Planning Trips with Girl Scouts."

Money Earning/Group Financing

Activities Involving Money

Girl Scout groups are financed by dues, money-earning activities, and a share of money earned through council-sponsored product sale activities. Daisy Girl Scouts may not be involved in raising or handling any money, including group dues and proceeds from group money-earning and product sale activities.

"Group money earning" refers to activities following a planned budget and carried out by girls and adults, in partnership, to earn money for the group treasury. "Council-sponsored product sale activities" are council-wide sales of authorized products, such as Girl Scout Cookies or calendars, in which groups participate. The funds are for Girl Scout activities and are not to be retained by individuals as their property.

Girls' participation in group money-earning projects or council-sponsored product sale activities is based on the following:

♦ Voluntary participation

♦ Written permission of a parent or guardian

♦ Council guidelines

♦ An understanding of and ability to interpret to others why the money is needed

♦ Correct business procedures

♦ Observance of local ordinances related to involvement of children in money-earning activities

♦ Adherence to guidelines for personal protection

♦ Planned arrangements for safeguarding the money

Girl Scouts, in their role as Girl Scouts, may not raise or solicit money for other organizations. However, girls may contribute a portion of their group treasury to organizations or projects they consider worthwhile if they have funds that are not needed for the activities during the year (for example, local or international community service organizations or environmental projects).

Encourage girls to designate a portion of their group treasury for the annual membership dues of the members. This is a sound and efficient practice that enables girls to meet membership dues and lessens the potential burden to individual members.

See activity checkpoints for "Girl Scout Cookie/Council-Sponsored Product Sale Activities," page 131.

See also Program Standards 29, 30, 31, 32 and 33.

 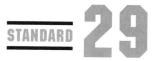

Group Money-Earning Activities

Money-earning activities are valuable program activities for girls. Daisy Girl Scouts do not participate in group money-earning activities.

Group leaders/advisors obtain written approval from their council before starting a group money-earning project. Money-earning activities may not be conducted on the Internet.

The number of money-earning projects may not exceed the amount of money needed to support group activities. The group determines the amount to be raised by preparing a group budget. Group money-earning activities need to be suited to the ages and abilities of the girls and consistent with the goals and principles of Girl Scout program. Review all procedures and equipment used to ensure that the activity is environmentally sound and the equipment is safe for girls to use. Some examples include making items and selling them; washing cars; putting on meals or dances for families; providing a gift-wrapping service; recycling beverage cans; working at special events in the community.

Product demonstration parties, raffles, drawings, games of chance, the

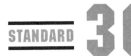

direct solicitation of cash, and the sale or endorsement of commercial products are examples of **inappropriate** money-earning activities.

Planning and participating in money-earning projects give girls the opportunity to learn many skills, such as budgeting, goal setting, customer relations, good business practices, and public relations.

Obtain the permission of a parent or guardian and make sure adults are present at all times when girls participate in money-earning activities outside their group meeting place.

The group submits a complete report on their money-earning activities, including an evaluation, to the council.

The income from group money-earning activities never becomes the property of individual members—girls or adults.

When girls are planning Girl Scout Gold Award projects or special service projects that require funds beyond the group treasury, they develop proposals that must be approved by the council before individuals or community businesses are solicited. The girls and an adult make the presentations to potential funders.

Council-Sponsored Product Sale Activities

Groups participate in no more than two council-sponsored product sale activities each year and only one of these may be a cookie sale. The percentage of money to be allocated to participating groups is determined by the council and explained to leaders prior to the product sale. Daisy Girl Scouts and their parents may not sell cookies or other products.

The selling of Girl Scout Cookies or other council-sponsored products is a valuable program experience for girls. These activities may not be conducted by adults. Adults serve in a supporting role for girls but should not assume sole responsibility for sales. Refer to the activity checkpoints for "Cookie/Council-Sponsored Product Sale Activities" on page 131.

Parents and guardians grant permission and are informed about the girls' whereabouts when they are engaged in product sales.

Girls should be identifiable as Girl Scouts by wearing a Membership Pin or uniform or carrying a membership card.

Adults must monitor, supervise, and guide the sale activities of all age levels. Brownie and Junior Girl Scouts must be accompanied by an adult. Girl Scouts 11 years of age or older-who participate in door-to-door sales must be supervised by an adult. Girls always use the buddy system.

Money due for sold products should be collected when the products are delivered or as directed by the Girl Scout council.

Girls may not engage in selling Girl Scout Cookies or other products approved for council-sponsored product sales on the Internet. Girls can use e-mail to let family and friends know about the sale.

Procedures for conducting council-sponsored product sales are determined by the council. The council provides training on the procedures to follow during the sale to all participants.

All girl members may participate in council-sponsored product sales activities. The council sets the guidelines for participation and determines how the proceeds and recognition system will be managed. The council retains some of the proceeds resulting from product sales to support program activities and participation of all registered Girl Scouts.

The income from product sales does not become the property of individual girl members.

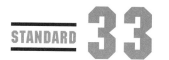 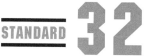

STANDARD 31

Council-Sponsored Product Sale Awards

Groups and individuals may choose to earn council product sale awards. Awards are program-related and of a type that will provide opportunities for girls to participate in Girl Scout activities.

Girls may earn the Girl Scout Cookie Sale Activity Pin as well as the age-appropriate award. In addition, each council may choose through a plan for recognition to provide items such as patches, camperships, event fees, day camp fees, scholarships for destinations, and materials and supplies for program activities to participants.

The council plan for recognition applies equally to all girls participating in the product sale activity.

STANDARD 32

Council Fund-Raising

Fund-raising or fund development to support the Girl Scout council is the responsibility of adults, and this responsibility should not be placed with girls. Girls may provide support to these efforts through voluntary service. Selling Girl Scout Cookies is not a fund-raising activity.

"Fund-raising" or "fund development" refers to any of various methods of soliciting contributed funds—for example, an annual campaign, a capital campaign, project funding, planned giving, benefits, and federated funds allocation.

Some examples of suitable ways for girls to support the council's fund-raising efforts include speaking about Girl Scout program, stuffing envelopes for an annual fund-raising campaign, assisting at a fund-raising function by carrying out a flag ceremony, escorting dignitaries, and putting together an audiovisual presentation.

STANDARD 33

Fund-Raising for Other Organizations

Girl Scouts, in their Girl Scout capacities, may not solicit money for other organizations. Girl members may support other organizations through service projects or a donation from their group treasury.

Some examples of suitable service projects to support other organizations include stuffing envelopes, delivering informational pamphlets to businesses, helping to organize and catalog books for a library book sale, serving as aides, or providing record-keeping assistance.

Girl Scouts, in their capacity as Girl Scouts, may not raise or solicit money for other organizations or participate in walkathons or telethons or similar activities that raise funds for other organizations. However, girls may contribute a portion of their group treasury to organizations or projects they consider worthwhile (for example, local or international community service organizations or environmental projects).

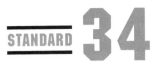

STANDARD 34

Collaborations with Other Organizations

Collaborative relationships or cooperative projects may be developed with other organizations whose goals and practices are compatible with Girl Scouting. All Girl Scout Program Standards are maintained during collaborative activities.

Obtain council approval before starting a cooperative project.

Brief organization representatives on all Girl Scout Program Standards, policies, and practices related to the project.

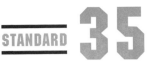

STANDARD 35

Political Activity

Girl Scouts, in their Girl Scout capacities, may not participate directly or indirectly in any political campaigns or participate in partisan efforts on behalf of or in opposition to a candidate for public office.

Girl Scouts are encouraged to become active and knowledgeable citizens, but must maintain a nonpartisan stand when acting in an official Girl Scout capacity. Wearing the uniform, citing a group number or council affiliation, or otherwise identifying oneself as a Girl Scout are examples of when one is acting in an official Girl Scout capacity.

Girl Scouts may express their opinions and beliefs when acting as individual citizens.

Letter-writing campaigns, circulating petitions, or carrying banners or signs at political rallies and functions are all examples of partisan political activity.

See the policy on political and legislative activity in the *Blue Book of Basic Documents.*

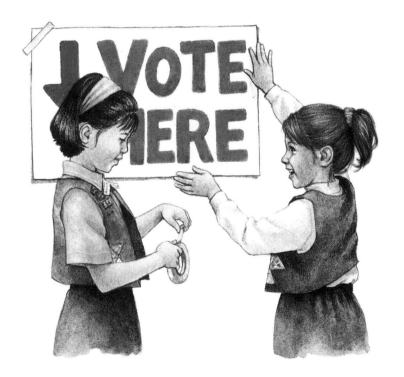

Activity Checkpoints

The checkpoints in this book guide the planning and implementation of specific activities. They represent the basic minimums to follow; they are not all-inclusive. They are the extensions of the basic safety guidelines and Program Standards in the preceding chapters and are also starting points for investigating resources with more in-depth information.

Three-Step Process

The process of preparing for an activity is organized into three steps:

1 In Step 1, the leader reads the planning checkpoints that are universally applied to all activities. They are general checkpoints that are considered before girls do any activity in Girl Scouting. See pages 81–83.

2 In Step 2, the leader/advisor reads the activity checkpoints that appear at the beginning of the chapter containing the activity that girls are planning. These activity checkpoints appear on pages 84, 94, and 112. They are general safety considerations that a leader/advisor always follows whenever the group does a particular type of activity such as camping, water sports, or land sports.

3 In Step 3, the leader/advisor studies the activity checkpoints for the particular activity of interest.

For example, a troop of Junior Girl Scouts would like to go ice skating. Their leader/advisor, having had council leadership training, reads the universal checkpoints on pages 81–83 and picks out items applicable to ice skating. She then turns to page 94 and reads the Step 2 checkpoints for Land Sports, and then turn to the specifics under Ice Skating.

Therefore, before beginning any activity, the leader/advisor must:

◆ Be familiar with all Program Standards and related guidelines.

◆ Review Steps 1, 2, and 3 in the activity checkpoints.

◆ Obtain written permission from parents or guardians, if necessary.

◆ Obtain council permission, if necessary.

◆ Refer to the Girl Scouts of the USA program resources for guidance. The handbooks for girls, leaders'/advisors' guides, and other supplemental resources contain activities carefully designed to bring the best possible experiences to girls.

Activities Not Listed in the Activity Checkpoints

When a group wants to plan an activity that is not listed in the activity checkpoints, use the following checklist to see if the activity is appropriate for Girl Scouting.

☐ Is the activity educationally sound?

☐ What are the overall benefits of the experience for the girls? Will the activity contribute to fulfilling the Program Goals accompanying Program Standard 1? (See page 63.)

☐ Is knowledgeable, trained, experienced leadership available to help the group plan and conduct the activity?

☐ What resources are required, including financial resources, equipment, and instruction?

☐ What are the potential health and safety risks and how will they be handled?

☐ Are the girls physically, emotionally, and intellectually ready?

☐ Is the activity a logical progression in skill building?

☐ What impact will there be on the environment?

☐ Is the site selected appropriate for the activity?

☐ Will council permission be required?

☐ Will additional parental permission be required?

☐ Will council insurance cover the activity?

In general, if an activity is not listed under one of the activity checkpoints or in another GSUSA publication, you should discuss the activity with the local council representative before making definite plans with the girls in your group.

Activities with High Risk

It is essential that the council be consulted if the proposed activity demands more physical prowess, emotional stamina, and greater skills than those listed in this book. Such activities may offer challenging experiences that promote girls' growth and development, but they also involve a wide range of variables that require extensive planning and expertise to control. With activities that require specialized skills, training, equipment, and supervision, care must be taken to control risks as much as possible as well as to ensure that participants are prepared for the activity and that the activity is conducted under optimum safety conditions. The skill and training required of participants and the leader or instructors must be carefully assessed and monitored.

If you receive council permission to conduct the activity, a set of activity checkpoints will be provided by the council. Make sure you, other adults involved in the activity, and the girls adhere to these checkpoints. Also, make an effort to reasonably accommodate any girls with special needs in the activity.

Some activities can carry a greater risk of severe injury or death even when they are conducted with great skill and care. There are also other considerations:

- Some may not be appropriate for certain age levels or persons of certain sizes.
- Some are harmful to the environment.
- Some are restricted by state law to persons of certain ages.
- Vendors who conduct some activities insist that contracts that hold the vendor harmless in case of an accident be signed by participants and/or their parents or guardians. A girl under the legal age of adulthood is not legally able to sign such an agreement or contract. Parents should be fully informed of their rights to sign or not sign such a contract. Any contracts or permission forms of this type should be reviewed by the council prior to entering into such arrangements.
- Other activities may not be currently insured by policies held by a particular Girl Scout council.

Therefore, it is necessary to check with your Girl Scout council before considering activities not listed in this book or other GSUSA resources.

Activities in the following list may not be attempted by a Girl Scout group without written authorization by their Girl Scout council. Girl Scout councils may not authorize any of these activities for girls under 12 years old and without ensuring that they are properly planned, supervised, and insured. Commercial operators or organizations that are insured and have professionally licensed or certified instructors for the particular activity should be chosen to conduct the activity rather than individuals who are not insured and licensed. Many of these activities may not be possible at all due to safety and insurance considerations in a particular area. Also, it may be necessary to cancel or postpone any planned activity due to extreme weather conditions or other unforeseen problems immediately prior to or during the conduct of the activity.

- Activities involving girls operating motorized vehicles such as go-carts and personal watercraft.
- Activities with uncontrollable and highly changeable environmental conditions such as watercraft trips on unclassified rivers.
- Activities that involve the use of firearms.
- Flights in noncommercial aircraft such as small private planes, helicopters, sailplanes, untethered hot air balloons, and blimps. The council must have liability insurance for non-owned aircraft in order to approve flights on any of these aircraft.

Activities That Are Not Permitted

The following are not permitted as Girl Scout program activities:

- Activities such as paintball that involve shooting a projectile at another person.
- Activities involving potentially uncontrolled free fall such as bungee jumping, hang gliding, parachuting, parasailing, and trampolining.
- Extreme variations of sports activities such as high altitude climbing and aerial tricks on bicycles, skis, snowboards, skateboards, and water skis.
- Hunting.
- Riding all-terrain vehicles and motor bikes.
- Watercraft trips in Class V and above whitewater.

Leaders or responsible adults with questions about the appropriateness of an activity should contact the council for guidance.

STEP 1

Universal Checkpoints

These checkpoints apply to every activity you do with girls in your role as a Girl Scout leader, volunteer, or staff member.

Council Approval

The leader/advisor:

☐ Keeps the Girl Scout council and parents and guardians informed about the activities of the girls.

☐ Obtains council approval for any activity that involves overnight travel, covers subjects of a sensitive or controversial nature, involves special equipment, or a money-earning project.

☐ Consults the council if uncertain whether a planned activity is in this category. Clearly describe the nature of the activity and, for activities that involve travel or special equipment, outline all the preparation, training, and safety precautions that are planned. Program Standard 15, on page 70, details the information that you need to give the council when seeking its approval.

☐ Discusses the activity with parents or guardians before including it in the group's plans.

☐ Gets council approval for specific activities, such as money-earning projects, certain types of service projects, and collaborations with other organizations.

Health

The leader/advisor:

☐ Reviews Program Standard 3. (See page 64.)

☐ Makes sure an annual health history is done for participation in physically demanding activities such as water sports, horseback riding, or skiing.

☐ Makes sure a health examination has been done within the preceding 24 months to participate in resident camping, in a trip of more than three nights, or in organized competitive sports. See page 39 for information on reducing the financial burden of a health examination.

Supervision

The leader/advisor:

☐ Makes sure instructors have certification from a recognized organization or equivalent certification, or have documented experience in the activity and meet any state or national qualification/certification requirements. See page 31 for information on documented experience.

☐ Ensures the appropriate girl–adult ratio and provides adequate and appropriate supervision.

Planning

The leader/advisor:

☐ Ensures that a girl isn't pushed beyond her capabilities. A girl's participation depends on her readiness: her level of maturity, physical conditioning, and level of training.

☐ Instructs or has girls instructed in basic and advanced skills as necessary.

☐ Provides adequate instruction with proper progression of skills.

☐ Reviews and practices safety rules.

☐ Has a ratio of adult supervisors to girls adequate for the degree of risk and the level of skill involved in the activity.

☐ Involves all participants in evaluating the activity.

☐ Is aware of each girl's ability. Schedules lessons and practice sessions for beginners that are conducted by qualified instructors.

Equipment and Clothing

The leader/advisor:

☐ Provides appropriate clothing, supplies, tools, and other equipment depending on the location and the specific activity. Communicates with parents and guardians of girls about the need for particular clothing or equipment for the activity.

Equipment

The leader/advisor:

☐ Is sure equipment is appropriate to the activity. Equipment suits a girl's age, size, maturity, experience, and ability, and is comfortable for her.

☐ Is sure equipment is in good working order and properly adjusted for each participant. Repairs or disposes of equipment that appears defective. Conducts a safety check of equipment prior to the activity.

☐ Uses safety equipment such as ropes, throw bags, and fire extinguishers that are appropriate to the activity. Makes sure it is easily accessible.

☐ Inspects rented or borrowed equipment carefully before using it. Rented or borrowed equipment, such as backpacks, skis, skates, and bicycles, should be selected, tested, and properly adjusted to suit each girl's size and ability.

☐ Ensures that protective eye safety equipment such as shatterproof lenses, eyeglass guards, or goggles are worn when appropriate in sports, arts and crafts, and science-related activities.

☐ Uses appropriate protective devices, such as safety helmets, in sports activities that require them. Safety helmets are designed to prevent injuries for a particular activity.

☐ Ensures that equipment regulated by legal standards meets the specified requirements. For example, all PFDs must be U.S. Coast Guard-approved, and all horseback riding helmets must meet the American Society for Testing and Materials (ASTM) standards.

☐ Reads and observes the manufacturer's instructions for safe use and care of equipment before use and keeps the instructions readily available. Safely stores all tools, equipment, and supplies (for example, power tools, paints, cleaning supplies, liquid fuels, and instruments with sharp edges) when not in use.

☐ Makes sure improperly equipped girls do not participate in the activity.

Clothing

The leader/advisor:

☐ Anticipates potential weather conditions and is prepared. Makes sure clothing and supplies protect against environmental hazards such as sunburn, heatstroke, and hypothermia. A protective lip balm will prevent chapped lips in all weather conditions. In sunny, hot weather, sunblocks and clothing covering shoulders and back will protect against sunburn. A number of thin layers provide better protection against cold than one heavy layer. A hat helps to retain body heat in the cold and protects against the sun in the heat. Wool clothing insulates well even when wet. Cotton breathes and absorbs moisture from the skin in hot weather but is not useful in cold, wet weather.

☐ Takes into account such factors as poisonous snakes and plants, bothersome insects and ticks.

☐ Suggests that uniforms are worn to provide identification for Girl Scouts traveling in groups, when appropriate.

☐ Suggests that loose-fitting clothing is worn to allow for freedom of movement during strenuous activity.

☐ Ensures that proper shoes and socks are worn to prevent fatigue, blisters, or general discomfort. Sturdy boots with thick soles

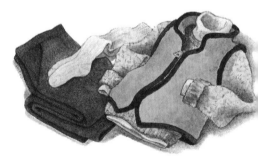

protect feet on rugged, rocky terrain and protect against bites from poisonous snakes.

☐ Is careful of dangling or flapping clothing that can be hazardous especially around playground equipment, bicycles, machinery with moving parts, or fires.

☐ Uses waterproof gear if there is a chance of getting wet, especially on cooler days when hypothermia is a concern.

Transportation

The leader/advisor:

☐ Makes arrangements in advance for all transportation and confirms plans before departure.

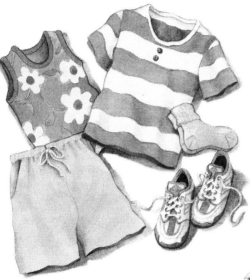

Site

The leader/advisor:

☐ Obtains council guidance and approval in selecting a site.

☐ Makes sure that a certificate of insurance for the facility is on file at the council office, if necessary.

☐ Is sure the facility is appropriate for the skills and ability levels of the girls.

☐ Is sure safety rules related to the specific activity are written, posted, understood, and practiced by all.

☐ Demonstrates respect for the environment.

☐ Monitors weather conditions.

☐ Inspects the site to be sure it is free of potential hazards.

Emergency Procedures and First Aid

The leader/advisor:

☐ Ensures that an adult with current first-aid training is present when required.

☐ Makes available first-aid equipment and supplies appropriate to the activity.

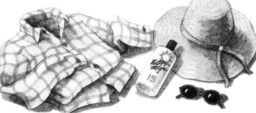

☐ Understands and practices first-aid procedures appropriate to the activity.

☐ Makes sure emergency medical care is accessible.

☐ Leaves an itinerary with a contact person at home. Calls the contact person upon departure and return.

☐ Writes and posts or carries a list of emergency telephone numbers.

☐ Reviews and is sure the group understands specialized safety and rescue procedures appropriate to the activity.

☐ Establishes security plans and procedures prior to activity participation. The leader, assisted by the girls, develops a security plan for the meeting place or activity area. Include procedures for determining the number of girls and their whereabouts at all times.

☐ Conducts a head count before and after every activity.

☐ Is sure every girl knows where to go and how to act when confronted by strangers or intruders and is able to sound an agreed-upon alarm.

CHAPTER 8
Camping Activities

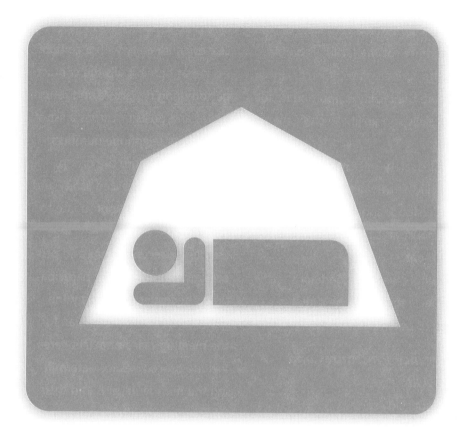

Before reading the next group of checkpoints, read those on pages 81–83, "Step 1: Universal Checkpoints."

Step 2
Activity Checkpoints

These checkpoints apply to all activities listed under the category "Camping Activities."

Planning and Supervision

The leader/advisor:

□ Uses the principles of minimal impact camping described in *Outdoor Education in Girl Scouting*.

□ Obtains site permits, if needed, in advance.

Equipment

The leader/advisor:

□ Uses flame-resistant tents. Plastic tents are not used.

□ Uses portable cookstoves whenever possible to reduce the use of wood in backcountry areas.

Clothing

The leader/advisor:

□ Makes a complete checklist of group and personal equipment and distributes it to group members.

□ Makes sure soft-soled shoes, such as sneakers, are worn around the campsite to reduce environmental impact. Girls learn the proper care of their feet, such as treatment for blisters.

Site

Campsite Sanitation

The leader/advisor:

☐ Stores garbage in an insect- and animal-proof container with a plastic inner lining, and covers it securely when there is a campsite garbage pickup service.

☐ When there is no garbage pickup service, removes all garbage from the campsite in plastic bags and discards as appropriate, or recycles whenever possible. Does not bury food. Carries out grease and fuel canisters.

Primitive Campsites

The leader/advisor:

☐ When primitive camping, chooses and sets up a campsite well before dark.

☐ Uses a previously established campsite if available.

☐ Makes sure the campsite is level and located at least 200 feet from all water sources and below tree-line.

☐ Avoids fragile mountain meadows and areas of wet soil.

☐ Avoids camping under dead tree limbs.

☐ Uses existing fire rings if a fire is necessary.

☐ If a latrine is not available, uses individual "cat holes"—at least 200 feet away from the trail and known water sources—to dispose of human waste.

☐ Does dishwashing and personal bathing at least 200 feet away from water sources.

☐ Stores food well away from tents and out of the reach of animals. Where necessary, hang food at least 10 feet high from a rope stretched between two trees. If the site is in bear country, check with local authorities on precautions to take.

☐ Sees that garbage, tampons, sanitary supplies, and toilet paper are carried out.

Emergency Procedures

The leader/advisor:

☐ Posts telephone numbers for all emergency care and council contacts where appropriate or the adult in charge carries them, and knows the location of the telephone.

☐ Writes, reviews, and practices evacuation and emergency plans for severe weather with girls and posts the plan.

Backpacking

Planning and Supervision

The leader/advisor:

☐ Takes council-approved training in backpacking.

☐ Plans and conducts a series of conditioning hikes before the backpacking trip.

☐ Determines the length of the trip by the backpackers' ages, their level of experience, their physical condition, the nature of the terrain, the weight of the load to be carried, the season and weather conditions, the water quantity and quality, and activities planned along the way.

☐ Ensures that the backpacking party consists of a minimum of four people, including two adults. One adult is in the lead and the other is at the rear of each group of backpackers. Ratios of girls to adults are consistent with the ratios for camping in Program Standard 13. (See page 69.)

☐ Ensures that backpackers have a comprehensive understanding of the trip. Group members are trained to be observant of the route, the surroundings, and the fatigue of individuals. Instruction is given on the safety rules for back-packing, such as staying together in a group, recognizing poisonous plants and biting or stinging insects and ticks, respecting wild animals, and behaving effectively in emergencies. Training is given in map reading, compass use, route navigation, and estimating distance.

☐ Ensures that a land management or similar agency is contacted during the trip planning stage to determine available routes and campsites, recommended group size, water quantity and quality, and permits needed.

☐ Checks that each girl carries at least one quart of water. There are adequate rest periods with time to replenish fluids and to eat high-energy foods.

☐ Develops guidelines for dealing with problems that may arise with other groups of backpackers.

Equipment

☐ Girls are given instruction on choosing backpacks, adjusting them, and taking them on and off.

☐ Backpacks and all equipment, food, and water being carried weigh no more than 20 percent of each person's ideal body weight.

☐ The foods taken are nutritious, nonperishable, high-energy, and easily digestible. Foods are packaged so as to reduce the number of containers and the amount of trash.

☐ Water purification supplies are carried. Water from all natural sources is considered potentially contaminated and is purified before drinking. Water filters designed to remove *Giardia lamblia* from water are used. (See "Outdoor Cooking," pages 89–91.)

Site

☐ The route is known to one of the adult leaders or a report is obtained in advance to assess potential hazards. The route chosen is within the ability of every girl in the group; the pace accommodates the slowest hiker.

☐ Hiking off-trail and after dusk is not permitted. The group hikes away from the edges of waterfalls, rock ledges, and slopes with loose rocks.

Emergency Procedures and First Aid

☐ A first-aider, level 2, is present.

☐ Methods of communication with sources of emergency care, such as police, hospitals, and park and fire officials, are known and arranged in advance.

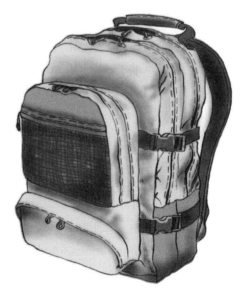

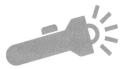

Group Camping

Planning and Supervision

☐ The leader/advisor has taken council group (troop) camp training in teaching and supervising group camping. As an alternative, a program consultant trained in group camping may help the leader and the girls prepare for the group camping trip and then accompany the leader and the group on the trip.

Group camp training generally covers these topics:

☐ Girl Scout program activities appropriate to the outdoor setting

☐ Discussion of other camping opportunities available to group members, including day, core-staff, and resident camp, as well as wider opportunities

☐ Group preparation for the trip, including procedures for cookouts, kapers, and special activities

☐ Activities and camping skills, including minimal impact camping skills, that represent steps in a natural progression

☐ Safety standards, activity checkpoints, supervision, and council policies for camping and outdoor activities

☐ The use of group government in camping

☐ Resources of the site and surrounding area

☐ First-aid and other emergency procedures

☐ Methods of dealing with homesickness

☐ Awareness and understanding of differing social, economic, and ethnic backgrounds

For group camping, the leader should also note the following:

☐ Each group is accompanied by at least two adults. The girl-to-leader ratios given in Program Standard 13 are observed. (See page 69.)

☐ Girls participate in the planning and preparation for the trip. Girls plan menus, activities, rules for group living, and on-site activities.

☐ Girls learn about appropriate clothing, footwear, bedding, packing, personal health care, and ways to dress for changes in weather conditions.

☐ Safety rules are observed for outdoor cooking, hiking, swimming, science activities, boating, etc. (Refer to the activity checkpoints for further information on these topics.)

Clothing

☐ Shoes, hiking boots, or sneakers and socks are worn; no sandals, flip-flops, or bare feet.

Equipment

☐ Sleeping bags are stuffed with filler appropriate for the anticipated temperature. (Check the label.)

☐ No candles, kerosene lamps, portable cookstoves, or any device with an open flame is ever used inside tents. Battery-powered lights are recommended. Lanterns fueled by propane, butane, kerosene, or gas may be used outdoors.

☐ Heaters may not be used inside tents.

Site

☐ State and local regulations related to drinking water, sanitation, fire building, etc., are observed.

☐ Before council approval, the site is inspected or a firsthand report is obtained in advance to assess any hazards and the suitability of the site.

☐ Potentially dangerous areas, such as sharp dropoffs, are clearly marked.

☐ Chemicals and flammable materials are locked in a dry, well-ventilated storage area.

☐ Fire extinguishers are available, suited to the activities, checked regularly, and accessible to all participants.

☐ Adults know how to use fire extinguishers.

☐ At least one toilet facility with an adjacent hand-washing facility is provided for every 20 overnight campers.

☐ Separate sleeping and bathroom facilities are provided for adult males accompanying the group.

☐ The site is left clean. "Clean" means removal of trash and evidence of human activities. It does not mean removal of natural materials, such as leaves, from trails.

☐ There is adequate shelter from possible inclement weather.

☐ Precautions are taken to protect against harmful insects and ticks, animals, and poisonous plants. Campers are taught to identify and avoid them.

☐ Mosquito netting and insect repellent are used where needed.

☐ Additional information can be found in *Outdoor Education in Girl Scouting.*

Emergency Procedures and First Aid

☐ A first-aider is present.

☐ A vehicle is available or an ambulance is on call at all times to transport an injured or sick person.

☐ Search-and-rescue procedures for missing persons are written out in advance, reviewed, and practiced by girls and leaders/advisors. The procedures are posted.

☐ A fire drill is practiced on the site, particularly from the sleeping area.

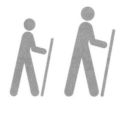

Hiking

This checkpoint does not apply to short walks.

Planning and Supervision

☐ Hikes are restricted to a reasonable length as determined by age, level of experience, nature of the terrain, physical condition of the hikers, disabilities, weather conditions, and time of day.

☐ The group leader/advisor has experience in teaching hiking techniques and trip planning.

☐ Instructions are given on the safety rules for hiking.

☐ The buddy system is used. The hiking party consists of a minimum of four people, including the adults. (If injury occurs, one person cares for the patient while the other two seek help.)

☐ There is one adult in the lead and another adult at the rear of each group of hikers.

☐ Girls are instructed in how to adjust day packs.

☐ Off-trail hiking is avoided. Girls stay on the pathway to avoid trampling trailside plants and causing erosion.

☐ Each girl carries a minimum of one quart of water.

☐ There are adequate rest periods, with time to replenish fluids and eat high-energy food.

☐ Guidelines are developed for dealing with problems that may arise with other groups of hikers.

Site

☐ The route is known to one of the adult leaders or a report is obtained in advance to assess potential hazards such as poisonous plants, dangerous animals, unsafe drinking water, cliffs, and dropoffs. Unsafe routes are avoided.

☐ The route chosen is within the ability of every girl in the group; the pace accommodates the slowest hiker.

☐ Terrain, mileage, and hiking time are known to the hikers in advance.

☐ Respect for the environment is demonstrated. Eating wild foods, walking on or uprooting plants, interfering with or feeding wild animals, and littering is avoided.

Emergency Procedures and First Aid

☐ A first-aider, level 1, is present. A first-aider, level 2, is present for hikes of 10 miles or more and away from emergency assistance.

☐ The first-aider is prepared to handle cases of hypothermia, blisters, sprains, fractures, insect stings and tick bites, snake bites, sunburn, and heat- and cold-related injuries.

☐ A search-and-rescue plan for lost hikers is written down and understood by everyone in advance.

National Organizations

Appalachian Mountain Club (www.outdoors.org), Appalachian Trail Conference (www.atconf.org).

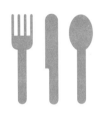

Outdoor Cooking

Planning and Supervision

☐ The leader/advisor supervising outdoor cooking has received council training.

☐ Girls should learn to use a variety of cooking methods, including use of propane, butane, and gas stoves, charcoal, "canned heat," and solar energy.

☐ The leader/advisor checks with the local fire district, land management agency, or conservation office to see whether a permit is required. Fires are not permitted when there is excessive dryness or wind. The leader also checks the fire index with local land management agencies or the fire district or consult the radio. Local air pollution regulations are followed.

☐ Girls are instructed in the food preparation and safe cooking skills listed in the tips below.

Clothing

☐ Cooks roll up long sleeves, tie back long hair, and do not wear plastic garments, such as ponchos, around an open flame.

Equipment

☐ Firefighting equipment is available, including fire extinguisher, water, loose soil or sand, and a shovel and a rake, as appropriate.

Emergency Procedures and First Aid

☐ Fire safety rules, emergency procedures, and first aid for burns are reviewed with the group and understood.

☐ Procedures are established and known in advance for notifying the fire department or land management agency officials in case of a fire.

☐ Fire drills are practiced at each site.

Portable Cookstoves

☐ Portable cookstoves differ in size and in fuel use. Follow the manufacturer's instructions carefully and closely supervise the girls when using any stove.

☐ Take an adequate amount of fuel. Store the extra fuel supply away from the cooking flame.

☐ Never use portable cookstoves inside a tent or indoors.

☐ Keep all stove parts clean. Check that lines and burners are not clogged.

☐ Do not refuel the cookstove or change canisters near an open flame. Take care not to spill fuel. If fuel does spill, relocate the stove before lighting it.

☐ Place portable cookstoves in safe, level, and stable positions, shielded from the wind and away from foot traffic.

☐ Do not pile rocks or other items around the cookstove for stability. Do not overheat the fuel tank.

☐ Use pots of appropriate size, so that the stove is not top-heavy.

☐ Store the extra fuel supply away from the cooking flame.

☐ Do not dispose of pressurized cans in a fire, place them in direct sunlight, or keep them in enclosed areas where the temperature is high. See the manufacturer's instructions on the label. Store and dispose of fuel canisters in the recommended manner.

Solar Stoves

☐ Remember that pots and food inside a solar oven are hot even if the stove does not feel hot. Use insulated gloves when removing the pot and opening the lid.

Open Fires

☐ Build fires in designated areas. Avoid establishing new fire sites, if possible. An established fire site is clear of overhanging branches, steep slopes, rotted stumps or logs, dry grass and leaves, and cleared of any burnable material, such as litter, duff, or pine needles.

☐ Where wood gathering is permitted, use only dead, fallen wood, and keep the cooking fires small.

☐ Store wood away from the fire area.

☐ Watch for flying sparks and put them out immediately.

☐ Before leaving the site, check that the fire is completely out: sprinkle the fire with water or smother it with earth or sand. Stir; then sprinkle or smother again. Finally, hold hands on coals, ashes, partially burned wood, or charcoal for one minute. It should be cool to the touch.

☐ Make a plan for disposing of cold ashes and partially burned wood. You may scatter ashes and burned wood throughout the woods away from the campsite.

☐ Do not put ashes and burned wood in a plastic pail; do not leave a pail with ashes or burned wood against the side of a building.

Charcoal Fires

☐ Charcoal fires are started with fuels explicitly labeled as charcoal starters—never use gasoline as a fire starter. Never add charcoal lighter fluid to a fire once it has started.

Tips for Food Preparation

☐ Meals are nutritionally sound, reflect girls' planning, and are prepared with consideration of food allergies, religious beliefs, and dietary restrictions of group members.

☐ Whenever possible, buy food and supplies that avoid excess packaging, and buy in bulk.

☐ Review health considerations, including the importance of keeping utensils, food preparation surfaces, and hands clean, cooking meats thoroughly, refrigerating perishables, and using clean water when preparing food. Do not use chipped or cracked cups and plates.

☐ Instruct girls in the safe use of kitchen tools and equipment, such as knives.

☐ Maintain discipline in the cooking area to prevent accidents with hot food and sharp utensils.

☐ Use long-handled cooking utensils and pot holders or insulated gloves to protect hands.

☐ Do not overfill cooking pots.

☐ Do not use pressurized cans, plastic basins, bottles, and cooking utensils near an open flame.

☐ No person with a skin infection, a cold, or a communicable disease participates in food preparation. Each person has an individual drinking cup.

Tips for Food Storage

☐ Store perishables such as creamed dishes, pudding, dairy products, poultry, meats, and salads at or below 45°F in a refrigerator or an insulated cooler with ice in it. If this is not possible, use powdered, dehydrated, freeze-dried, or canned foods.

☐ On extended trips, do not use foods requiring refrigeration.

☐ Use safe water to reconstitute powdered, dehydrated, or freeze-dried food. Once reconstituted, eat perishable items within one hour or refrigerate them.

Water Purification Tips

☐ Access a safe drinking water supply for cooking, drinking, and personal use. Safe drinking water is defined as tap water tested and approved by the local health department. All other sources are considered potentially contaminated and must be purified before use. *Giardia lamblia* is suspected in all surface water supplies. There are three ways to purify water.

First, strain water through a clean cloth into a clean container to remove sediment and then choose one of the following methods:

1. Boil water rapidly for a full minute and let it cool.

2. Disinfect water with water purification tablets, following the manufacturer's instructions. Check the shelf life of the product to make sure it has not expired.

3. Pour water through a specially designed water filtration device that is designed to remove *Giardia*. These filters will also remove many other contaminants. Follow the manufacturer's instructions carefully.

Note that only boiling the water or pouring it through a specially designed filter will remove *Giardia lamblia*. These methods will not remove chemical pollutants.

Dishwashing Tips

☐ Wash dishes in a prescribed area according to this procedure:

☐ Remove food particles from utensils and dishes.

☐ Wash dishes in warm, soapy water.

☐ Rinse dishes in hot, clear water.

☐ Sanitize dishes by rinsing in clear, boiling water or immersing for at least one minute in a sanitizing solution approved by the local health department.

☐ Air-dry and store dishes in a clean, covered area.

☐ Dispose of dishwashing and rinse water according to the campsite regulations. In backcountry areas, dispose of wastewater on the ground at least 200 feet beyond any water source or trail.

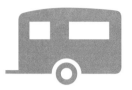

Trip/Travel Camping

Experienced campers—girls and adult leaders—can plan and go trip camping. Trip camping involves camping at different sites over three or more nights and traveling from one site to another under one's own power or by vehicle or animal that permits individual guidance (for example, bicycle, canoe, horse, sailboat).

Travel camping (using campsites as a means of accommodations) is planned and carried out by a group of girls and adult leaders who are experienced campers. The group uses motorized transportation to move from one site to another over a period of three or more nights. Motorized transportation is usually a bus, van, or automobile but may also be an airplane, boat, or train, or a combination of vehicles.

Planning and Supervision

When preparing for and conducting the trip, use the activity checkpoints in this book; specifically, check the mode of travel (canoeing, backpacking, kayaking, bicycling, skiing) and the activities engaged in (such as outdoor cooking or swimming).

☐ The trip/travel camping leader possesses knowledge, skills, and experience in the following areas:
- Outdoor leadership
- Progression and readiness
- Trip planning
- Safety management
- First aid, safety, handling emergency situations
- Judgment and maturity
- Program activities specific to the trip
- Group dynamics and management
- Supervision of both girls and adults
- Participation in similar trips
- Familiarity with the area in which the trip is conducted
- Physical fitness and skills necessary to lead the group

☐ A minimum of two adult leaders/advisors, at least one of whom is female, are present on each trip. In addition, follow the adult-to-girl ratio as set in Program Standard 13. (See page 69.)

☐ Adult leaders selected for the trip are trained or have documented experience in the following areas:
- Travel or trip camping skills
- Group management and group dynamics
- Child development
- Mode of transportation
- Site orientation
- First aid and cardiopulmonary resuscitation (CPR)
- Emergency procedures
- Operational procedures
- Minor maintenance for equipment and vehicle, as appropriate

☐ For each trip, girls and leaders receive a pre-trip orientation that includes the following:
- First-aid procedures
- Use of the buddy system and emergency and rescue procedures
- Environmental awareness and protection procedures
- Program plans for mode of travel and geographic area
- Operational procedures: purification of water, food preparation, camping equipment, sanitation procedures, and food storage procedures

☐ For trips by small craft, the supervising adult is currently certified as an instructor as specified in the activity checkpoint for the particular mode of transportation or certified in Small Craft Safety from the American Red Cross, or has equivalent certification or documented experience indicating knowledge and skill in the supervision of similar trips.

☐ For trips that involve swimming, an adult currently certified in lifeguarding or the equivalent is present.

☐ A currently signed agreement with providers of trip/travel camping services specifies responsibility for compliance with these trip/travel camping guidelines.

Equipment

☐ Girls and adult leaders/advisors are protected from the natural elements (rain, snow, wind, sun, cold, insects, ticks, etc.) by the following, as appropriate to the geographic location and season:

- Shelter
- Clothing
- Sleeping gear
- Repellents
- Sunblocks

☐ Each girl and leader/advisor wears an identifying bracelet or similar device with the following information on it:

- Name of girl or adult
- Name of Girl Scout council
- Telephone number of emergency contact

☐ All girls and adult leaders/advisors have on their person a card with their name, address, and telephone number; the council name, address, and telephone number; and the name of a contact person.

Transportation

☐ Each driver of motorized transportation is at least 21 years old and holds a valid operator's license appropriate to the vehicle. The Girl Scout council checks the operator's driving record.

☐ There is a relief driver for trips of more than four hours. The relief driver holds a valid operator's license for the vehicle operated, and her or his driving record is checked.

☐ If a trailer is used, it is in compliance with all state, local, and federal regulations for the areas of travel. The assigned driver is experienced in pulling a trailer. No girls or adult leaders ride in the trailer.

Emergency Procedures and First Aid

☐ A first-aider, level 2, is present.

☐ There are written procedures to follow if a group member needs to be removed from the trip.

☐ The group communicates with the contact person at home or the council office about the progress of the trip.

☐ Phone numbers and exact locations of medical assistance and emergency help are carried on the trip. A copy of the complete trip plan is on file with the council office.

CHAPTER 9
Land Sports

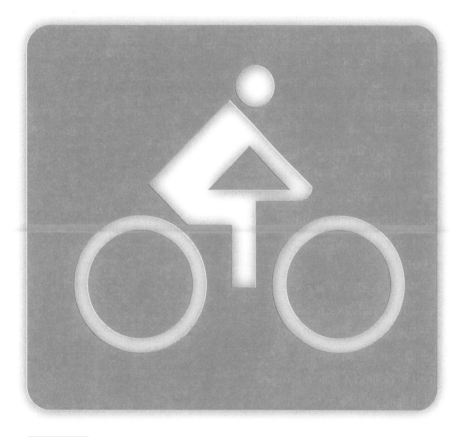

Activity Checkpoints

Read the Step 1 checkpoints on page 81 and these Step 2 checkpoints before reading the checkpoints in this chapter.

Planning and Supervision

The leader/advisor:

☐ Makes sure instructors have thorough knowledge of safety practices, equipment use and maintenance, and technique.

☐ Reviews the rules and operating procedures with the girls before each session.

☐ Makes sure the safety rules are written, understood, practiced, and posted at the site.

Equipment

The leader/advisor:

☐ Secures all equipment in a dry, locked storage area.

Clothing

The leader/advisor:

☐ Makes sure girls and adults avoid wearing jewelry, especially pierced earrings, looped earrings, bracelets, and necklaces in contact sports or where jewelry may become entangled in equipment.

Emergency Procedures and First Aid

The leader/advisor:

☐ Makes sure a list of emergency telephone numbers, including those for emergency rescue services and the police, is posted or carried by the adult in charge.

□ Teaches girls to take shelter away from tall objects in a storm with lightning and thunder. Find the lowest point in an open flat area. Squat low to the ground on the balls of the feet. Have girls place their hands on their knees with their heads between them. Instruct girls to make themselves the smallest targets possible and to minimize their contact with the ground.

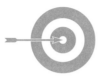

Archery

Archery is not recommended for Daisy or Brownie Girl Scouts. A participant in archery activities must be old enough to understand safety procedures and handle equipment so as not to endanger herself, other participants, or onlookers.

Planning and Supervision

□ One adult is a currently certified National Archery Association instructor or has equivalent certification or documented experience indicating knowledge and skill in teaching/supervising archery.

□ A ratio of 1 to 10 participants to each instructor is observed.

□ A whistle system for starting, retrieving, and emergency stopping is in effect.

□ Girls develop skills based on proper procedures and form, such as stringing the bow, nocking the arrow, stance, sighting, and observing safety practices.

□ Archers straddle the shooting line to shoot.

□ Girls waiting to shoot are behind the shooting line.

□ A ground quiver for arrows is provided for each line of shooters.

□ Archery games away from a regular course are well supervised and appropriate to age, skill level, and location of shooting.

Equipment

□ Bows and arrows are appropriate to the age, size, strength, and ability of the girls.

□ Girls have finger and arm protection, such as finger tabs and arm guards. Right- and left-handed models are available.

□ Arrows are not warped and do not have cracked nocks or loose or missing feathers.

□ Bowstrings do not have broken or loose strands.

□ Bows do not have loose or broken arrow rests.

□ Backstops for targets are in good repair.

□ A beginner uses arrows that extend one to two inches in front of the bow when the bow is at full draw. Only target tip arrows are used, never broadhead tips.

Transportation

□ Provisions are made for safe handling of archery equipment to and from the range.

Site

For an Outdoor Range

☐ Targets are not placed in front of houses, roads, trails, or tents. Avoid areas with any pedestrian traffic. Clear areas of brush. A hillside backstop is preferable.

☐ The shooting area and the spectator area behind the shooting area are clearly marked.

☐ In the shooting area, there is a distance of at least 50 yards behind the targets and 20 yards on each side of the range.

☐ An outdoor range is not used after nightfall.

For an Indoor Range

☐ An indoor range shooting distance is a maximum of 20 yards.

☐ Targets are well lighted.

☐ Doors or entries onto the range are locked or blocked from the inside. (Do not block fire exits.)

National Organizations

National Field Archery Association (www.nfaa-archery.org).

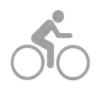

Bicycling

Bicycles are the proper size and in good condition. Each bike is thoroughly checked before any day or extended trip.

Planning and Supervision

☐ Instruction is given by an adult with experience, knowledge, and skill in teaching and/or supervising bicycling.

☐ Girls are instructed in and practice bicycle-riding skills in traffic, including signaling, scanning ahead and behind (especially before moving left), yielding to oncoming traffic, and making left turns.

☐ The length and terrain of a trip, day or extended, are appropriate to the girls' skill level, their experience, and their physical condition, as well as the time of day, the weather, and the equipment available.

☐ Following are some general tips for preparing for a trip and being on the road:

■ Obtain bike route maps or lists of recommended bike routes that many states publish.

■ Obtain bicycle licenses where required (some localities license the bike, not the cyclist).

■ Review the route and practice map-reading skills before departure. Be sure to take the map.

■ Make careful plans for the type of road to be traveled. For example, secondary roads are quiet, but may have trees, curves, and hills that obstruct visibility.

■ Ride bicycles only during daylight hours.

☐ Participants are taught to recognize and avoid common hazards, including vertical drain grates, sand, gravel, glass, wet leaves, and litter on shoulders, and other road-surface hazards, to communicate and cooperate with other road users, and to ride defensively. Motor vehicle traffic presents the greatest danger to cyclists; hazards such as oil, wet leaves, parked cars, and rocks cause the majority of cycling accidents.

☐ Participants practice bicycling with a load comparable in weight to the load on the trip.

☐ Participants learn to brake before they have to, especially on curves and downhills. Emergency braking techniques are taught.

☐ Participants cycle single file with traffic; it is acceptable to ride briefly two abreast when passing a slower bicyclist.

☐ Except when on bicycle paths, participants travel in groups of five or six, allowing at least 150 feet between groups so that vehicles may pass.

□ Participants ride one to a bicycle except when riding tandem. In tandem riding, each girl has her own seat and the number of riders doesn't exceed the intended limits of the bicycle.

□ For every two groups, there is an adult at the head and another at the rear.

□ Participants ride with the flow of traffic and obey applicable traffic regulations, signals, lane markings, and local ordinances pertaining to bicycle operation.

□ Bicyclists do not weave in and out of traffic or between parked cars.

□ Light gear is stored in bicycle panniers or packs on the back of the bike.

□ Bicyclists make a full stop and look left, right, and left again, especially at the end of a driveway, before entering a street or roadway.

□ Bicycles are walked across busy intersections.

□ Bicyclists use hand signals to indicate turning or stopping.

□ Bicyclists keep a safe distance between themselves and the vehicle ahead.

□ Bicycles have lights and reflectors. When bicycles are not on segregated bicycle paths, lights are on to increase visibility.

Clothing

□ Participants wear comfortable, close-fitting clothing that cannot catch in the gears or the chain; they use pant clips or bands if needed.

□ Participants wear reflective or very light colored clothes when cycling at dusk.

□ Participants wear bright colored or fluorescent clothing during the day.

□ Participants wear layers of clothing on extended trips and carry extra clothes and rain gear.

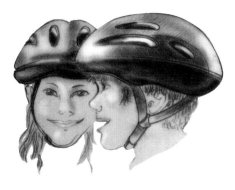

The helmet should be worn level on the head. It should not move in any direction when the chin strap is securely fastened.

Equipment

□ Bicycle helmets are worn to prevent head injuries. Purchase helmets that meet the Consumer Product Safety Commission standard.

□ Helmets are sized properly to fit comfortably but snugly.

□ Each bicycle group carries a repair kit containing a pump, a tire patch kit, tire irons, a screwdriver, an adjustable wrench, pliers, and lubricating fluids.

□ Each bike is in working order, including horn or bell, headlamp, taillight, and reflectors.

Site

□ Observe all state and local regulations.

□ Use designated bicycle trails whenever possible.

□ Select bicycle trails with even surfaces.

□ Avoid routes involving heavily traveled streets and highways.

□ Notify jurisdictional authorities about the group's trip, when necessary.

□ Know the location of emergency and medical services along the route in advance.

Emergency Procedures and First Aid

□ A first-aider is present.

□ Provide a detailed itinerary and an established call-in schedule for each day.

□ Carry a list of emergency phone numbers and addresses of bike repair shops.

□ Carry identification at all times.

□ Be capable of emergency maneuvers (for example, panic stop, rock dodge, instant turn).

Additional Checkpoints for Bicycle Touring

☐ Conditioning your body before the tour is important. Long-distance, overnight touring can involve many hours of cycling, sometimes in difficult terrain and with more weight than on day trips.

☐ Adjust bicycles frequently for comfort. Check the handlebars after adjusting the seat for proper leg extension.

☐ Use padded handlebars or wear cycling gloves to soften road vibrations.

☐ Carry two or three water bottles each and drink frequently. Avoid carbonated beverages.

☐ Do not stop cycling abruptly. After stopping, cool down gradually by walking around for a few minutes.

☐ Learn to listen to your body and do not push past your endurance level.

National Organizations

Bicycling Federation of America (www.bikefed.org), Hostelling International—American Youth Hostels (www.hiayh.org), National Safety Council (www.nsc.org).

Caving

Caving is not done by Daisy or Brownie Girl Scouts. This activity checkpoint also does not apply to groups taking trips to tourist caves, such as Carlsbad Caverns.

Cavers must understand safety procedures and know how to handle equipment. Girls receive basic guidelines about caving before planning a caving trip.

Planning and Supervision

☐ A guide with documented experience in cave exploration accompanies the group into the cave. A guide can also help decide which caves are suitable.

☐ Pretrip instruction is given by an adult with documented experience indicating knowledge and skill in teaching and/or supervising caving.

☐ Each group has a minimum of five and a maximum of 10 people, including two adults. One adult is an experienced caver.

☐ In wet weather, caves with stream passages are avoided. Some caves can flood.

Clothing

Each person has:

☐ Sturdy boots with good ankle protection

☐ Gloves

☐ Kneepads (as needed)

Equipment

Each person has:

☐ A safety helmet that fits properly, with a strong chin strap. For horizontal caves, bump helmets may be used. For vertical caves, use safety helmets carrying the Union of International Alpine Association (UIAA) seal, which is located on the inside of the helmet.

☐ Three sources of light. The main light is electric and mounted on the safety helmet. The other two light sources may be flashlights.

☐ Food.

☐ Water.

☐ Trash bag. (Use as a poncho or for dirty equipment after the trip. Cavers keep an empty trash bag in their safety helmet.)

☐ Spare bulbs and batteries.

Site

☐ Obtain guidance from a local chapter of the National Speleological Society to select a cave to explore. Never explore a cave without a guide and written permission from the site owner/operator.

Emergency Procedures and First Aid

☐ A first-aider is present.

☐ The group leader carries the names and telephone numbers of the local cave rescue unit and rescue squad. These numbers are taped inside the leader's safety helmet. A second responsible adult carries a backup list.

☐ In the event of serious injury, at least two people stay with the injured person and two others seek help.

☐ Advance arrangements are made for medical emergencies and evacuation procedures.

National Organization

National Speleological Society (www.caves.org).

Challenge Courses, Climbing, and Rappelling

Challenge Courses (Initiative Games and Low Ropes and High Ropes Courses)

A challenge course is a set of structures that provide a setting for physical challenges designed to increase participant self-confidence and physical coordination, to increase group cooperation, and to have fun. They may be set up as initiative games, low elements, or high elements with a progression that teaches group trust, communication skills, muscle warm-up and stretching activities, and group challenges.

Each participant must possess the physical strength and technical skills to use the equipment, and understand the safety procedures and consequences of her action. A safety belay is used whenever the participant is on a structure more than six feet off the ground.

Initiative games and low elements require the group to work together to accomplish mental or physical challenges. Low ropes courses are not recommended for Daisy Girl Scouts.

High ropes courses involve components for individual or group challenges that are six feet or more off the ground. A safety belay is used with a harness, and a helmet is worn by the participants. High ropes courses are not recommended for Daisy and Brownie Girl Scouts.

Climbing

Girls may participate in three types of climbing:

☐ Bouldering. Climbing without a rope but at a height not greater than six feet off the ground. Spotters are used. Spotting is a safety system in which participants safeguard the movements of a member of the group. Spotters provide support and protect the head and upper body of a climber in case of a fall. Spotting is used on low elements of a challenge course, descending and ascending high elements or climbing routes, and bouldering.

☐ Top roping. A climbing method in which the climb is anchored from the top of the climbing route. The belayer may be set up at the top or the bottom of the route.

☐ Multi-pitch climbing (for experienced climbers only). A climb on a long route that requires several pitches the length of the rope or less. The climbing group all climb to the top of the first pitch. The lead climber climbs the next pitch, anchors in, and belays each remaining climber individually to the anchor.

Climbing may be done on indoor or outdoor artificial climbing walls, climbing/rappelling towers, and natural rock.

Rappelling

Rappelling is a means of descending by sliding down a rope. The rope runs through a mechanical device. A safety belay is used in all rappelling activities. Rappelling is not recommended for Daisy and Brownie Girl Scouts.

Planning and Supervision

☐ An instructor with documented experience, indicating competence in equipment maintenance, safety and rescue techniques, group processing techniques, proper use of the course and hands-on training directly supervises the group. The instructor has provided written documentation of the completed training.

☐ There is a regular process of review and update for all instructors.

☐ A minimum of two instructors are present.

☐ The instructor/participant ratios are as follow:

Challenge Courses:
- Low elements—1 instructor to 10 participants
- High ropes with dynamic belay—1 instructor to 10 participants
- High ropes with static belay—1 instructor to 7 participants

Bouldering, top roping, and indoor climbing walls—1 instructor to 10 participants

Multi-pitch climbing—1 instructor (qualified lead climber) to 3 participants

☐ Instructors are skilled in selecting appropriate activities, teaching and supervising spotting and belaying techniques and modifying tasks to provide an appropriate experience for the ages and skill levels in the group.

☐ Before use, instructors inspect all equipment, course components, and landing areas in the activity area.

☐ A set of readiness and action commands are taught to all participants for climbing, spotting, and belaying.

☐ All participants utilize muscle warm-up and stretching activities before beginning physical activities.

☐ Instructors describe the objectives, safety procedures, and hazards to the participants before beginning an activity. A debriefing follows the activity.

☐ Spotting techniques are taught, demonstrated, and practiced by participants prior to any climbing/challenge course activity. All activities are appropriately spotted.

☐ For activities where partners are needed, instructors match participants according to size and skill level, if appropriate.

☐ Instructors supervise all tie-ins, belays, and climbs on the high ropes course and climbing sites and spotting on the low elements course and bouldering sites.

☐ Participants are not stacked more than three levels high vertically (in a pyramid, for example) on each other at any time. No one should stand in the middle of someone else's back.

Equipment

☐ All equipment used for belaying—ropes, webbing, harnesses, hardware, helmets—is designed, tested, and manufactured for the purpose of this type of activity and appropriate for the size of the user. A chest harness with seat harness or full body harness is recommended for younger girls when climbing.

☐ Climbing helmets that have the UIAA-approved label (Union of International Alpine Association) must be worn for all climbing situations where the participant is

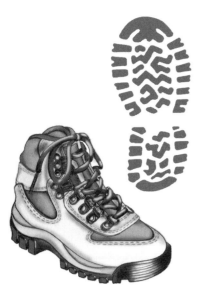

more than six feet off the ground. This includes outdoor climbing, bouldering, rappelling, and high ropes on challenge courses. They are not needed indoors unless required by the facility operator. It is recommended that a disposable liner, such as a shower cap or surgical cap, be worn underneath the helmet to protect against the spread of head lice.

☐ Participants on multi-pitch climbing routes carry their own water, sunscreen, raingear, food, and clothing appropriate for the weather conditions.

☐ There is a documented maintenance schedule and periodic inspection of all artificial structures and equipment used in the activities by instructors and outside professionals. A use log is kept on all equipment subject to stress, wear and deterioration. A written equipment monitoring and retirement

process is established and followed. The records are retained.

Clothing

☐ All instructors and participants wear sturdy shoes. Long pants are recommended for activities when skin abrasions on legs are possible (i.e., going over a log or wall on a challenge course). Loose clothing, especially around the head and neck, should be avoided.

☐ All sharp objects, jewelry, and watches should be removed and pockets emptied. Long hair is pulled back from the face and fastened under the helmet to prevent tangling.

Site

☐ Permits and permission requests are filed as required for climbing sites and facilities.

☐ All permanent structures and the belaying system are planned and constructed by experienced individuals.

☐ Plans and procedures are established to avoid unauthorized use of the site, structures, and equipment. The artificial climbing site and challenge courses site must be posted to warn against unauthorized use.

☐ When climbing and rappelling in natural areas, clean climbing techniques are taught and practiced.

Emergency Procedures and First Aid

☐ A first-aider, level 1, is present. A first-aider, level 2, is present for high ropes courses and multi-pitch climbing.

☐ A first-aid kit is available along with rescue equipment appropriate to the activity.

☐ On natural rock climbs, a climbing plan, including an alternate route, if appropriate, is filed with local authorities and a back-home contact. The authorities and the back-home contact person are notified upon departure and return. Be prepared to alter the climbing plan if weather conditions change.

☐ Specialized safety and rescue procedures are planned and practiced to ensure the ability to remove a participant from a high ropes, rappelling, or climbing situation. A sharp knife, hardware, and extra rope of appropriate length for rescue is available at the site.

☐ Emergency transportation is available.

National Organizations

Association for Experiential Education (www.aee.org), Association for Challenge Course Technology.

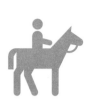

Horseback Riding

Horseback riding is not recommended for Daisy Girl Scouts. Daisy Girl Scouts may participate in pony rides when the animals are led by persons on foot.

Girls must possess sufficient physical coordination and balance to participate in riding. They are old enough to understand and practice safety procedures, to use good judgment in reacting to situations, and to take responsibility for themselves and their horses. (Some stables have weight limits for rider eligibility. Check when making reservations.)

Planning and Supervision

- ☐ Riding instructors are adults who have current certification from an accredited horsemanship instructor training organization or documented proof of a minimum of three years' experience successfully instructing in a general horseback riding program.
- ☐ Assistant riding instructors are at least 16 years old and are currently certified by an accredited horsemanship instructor training organization or have documented proof

of at least one year's experience successfully instructing in a general horseback riding program.

- ☐ Riders are supervised by instructors or assistant instructors at all times when in the proximity of horses, whether mounted or not.
- ☐ Each rider is tested and classified according to her riding ability. The horse and the riding area are assigned according to the rider's ability.
- ☐ Beginning riders attend an introductory safety lesson, including information on horse psychology and behavior and approaching, handling, and leading a horse.
- ☐ Before trail riding, a beginning rider rides in a ring or a corral. Riders must feel confident and demonstrate basic skills in controlling the horse (stop, start, and steer) and maintaining proper distance.
- ☐ An instructor makes a safety check of each rider's clothing, footwear, and helmet, the horse's tack, and the riding area before each riding session.
- ☐ Only one rider is allowed on a horse at any time.
- ☐ There is no eating or drinking while riding.

Additional Checkpoints for Ring or Corral Riding

- ☐ At least one instructor and one assistant instructor supervise a group of 10 or fewer riders, with one additional instructor or assistant instructor for every five additional riders.
- ☐ A pre-ride demonstration is given to all first-time riders, including mounting, dismounting, starting, stopping, steering, and maintaining a balanced body position.
- ☐ Each horse and rider is under the observation of an instructor at all times.
- ☐ The riding ring has good footing for the horses and is free of dangerous obstructions. The fencing is at least 42 inches high, visible, and well maintained. Gates to the ring are shut.

Additional Checkpoints for Trail Riding

- ☐ Each group is limited to no more than 10 riders, excluding an instructor and assistant instructor. For beginning riders or younger girls, or for difficult trails, increased supervision may be needed.
- ☐ The length of the trail ride and the gait of the horses are geared to the ability of the least experienced rider.
- ☐ Riding trails have good footing and are free of dangerous obstructions such as low-hanging branches.

- ☐ Trails are marked, mapped, regularly inspected, and maintained.
- ☐ Equipment for a trail ride includes helmets, halters, lead ropes, and rain gear.
- ☐ Gates are left as found, open or shut.
- ☐ Gear and first-aid kit are tied to the saddle or packed in saddlebags. Riders do not wear backpacks, day packs, fanny packs, etc.
- ☐ Before the trail ride, riders warm up in a ring or corral to ensure that they are well suited to their horses and can control all the gaits and functions required during the trail ride.
- ☐ The participants ride single file, one full horse length apart, with an instructor at the head and at the rear of the group.
- ☐ Riders have control of their horses, maintain the spacing between horses, and increase distances between horses when the horses' speed increases.
- ☐ Public roads and highways are avoided whenever possible. (If a group must cross a road, the instructor first halts the group in a line well before the road, checks for traffic, and then signals the group to cross. At the signal, all horses are turned to face the highway and all cross at the same time.)

- ☐ Horses are walked up and down hills, and for the final 10 minutes of any riding period in order to cool down.

Other Situations

- ☐ In other riding situations, such as open range riding, horse shows, or parades, a written safety management plan specific to the activity is prepared.
- ☐ Some activities, such as riding for girls with disabilities, vaulting, pack trips, driving, and games, may require special equipment, as well as horses and instructors with specialized training.

Clothing

- ☐ Long pants and appropriate protective clothing are worn. Clothing is snug to prevent tangling with the saddle.
- ☐ Boots or shoes with a smooth sole and at least a half-inch heel are worn to prevent feet from sliding through the stirrups.
- ☐ If tappaderos (a covering across the front of the stirrup that holds the foot in) are used, an athletic shoe with a nonskid sole may be worn.
- ☐ Riders may not ride barefoot, in sandals, or in hiking boots with lug soles.
- ☐ Riders may wear well-fitting gloves to protect hands from blisters, rope burns, and cuts.

Equipment

- ☐ Protective headgear with a properly fitting safety harness that meets the American Society for Testing and Materials (ASTM) F-1163-88 requirements, displaying the Safety Equipment Institute (SEI) seal, is worn by girls and adults, including all instructors, wranglers, stable hands, etc., while riding and preparing to ride.
- ☐ Equipment is properly adjusted for each rider and horse.
- ☐ Saddle size is appropriate for each rider.
- ☐ Girth straps are fitted properly and checked by the instructor prior to mounting and throughout mounted sessions.
- ☐ Stirrup lengths are adjusted for each rider.

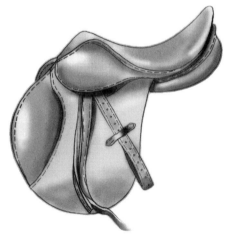

Site

- ☐ The stable operator provides evidence of liability insurance and instructor certification and references from other youth group users of the stable.
- ☐ For both Girl Scout council and non-Girl Scout riding facilities:
- ☐ The riding area is away from outside distractions and free of debris.
- ☐ The barn and riding areas do not have exposed barbed wire fencing.
- ☐ The instructional rings, corrals, paddocks, and stables have clearly posted rules and regulations.
- ☐ The horses are properly cared for, and the stables, corrals, barns, etc., are clean and uncluttered.
- ☐ Tack (saddles, bridles, etc.) is clean and in good condition.
- ☐ Weather conditions are suitable for riding. The ground is firm and free of ice.
- ☐ Riding is done during daylight hours only. Riding at night is in an enclosed, well-lighted area.
- ☐ Permission and any necessary permits are obtained before riding on public or private lands.
- ☐ Records of maintenance checks, requests, and repairs are kept.

Emergency Procedures and First Aid

- ☐ A first-aider, level 1, is present.
- ☐ An emergency vehicle is readily available.
- ☐ Plans for communication with emergency services and fire officials are arranged in advance and known by each instructor.
- ☐ Plans for response in an emergency, such as a fire, severe weather, an injured rider, an injured or loose horse, etc., are known by all participants and instructors.
- ☐ At Girl Scout facilities, communication between the riding area and the site director or health care personnel is possible.
- ☐ In stable and ring areas, telephone numbers for the fire department, local hospital or emergency ambulance service, and veterinarian are conspicuously posted, and the location of the fire alarm is known to all girls and adults.

National Organizations

Certified Horsemanship Association (CHA), Horsemanship Safety Association, Inc., United States Pony Club (www.ponyclub.org).

Ice Skating

Planning and Supervision

Ice Skating Rink

- ☐ The rink supervisor is called in advance to arrange for large groups or for practice sessions. (Check with the rink supervisor in advance to learn how many adults, in addition to the rink staff, are needed to supervise the group.)
- ☐ Leaders supervise from outside the main skating floor.
- ☐ An experienced ice skating instructor instructs girls in basic ice skating skills, safety, and conduct rules. Practice sessions are scheduled for beginners.
- ☐ Girls learn to perform basic skating skills, including how to fall and get up, before attempting more advanced skills.
- ☐ Warm-up exercises are done before any strenuous ice skating; cool-down exercises end the sessions.
- ☐ The rules of the rink are observed. For example:
  - Everyone skates in the same direction.
  - Girls do not stop in the main skating area.
  - Skaters yield the right-of-way to those already in the rink.

- Skaters do not cut across the paths of other skaters.
- Skaters do not push, shove, or race on the ice.
- A falling skater does not grab hold of another skater.
- A fallen skater rises quickly, unless injured.

☐ Loose or sharp articles, such as handbags, combs, and keys are not carried in pockets, hands, hair, or anyplace where they might cause injury to the skater in the event of a fall, or injure another skater by falling to the floor.

Outdoor Ice Skating

☐ Girls skate on a pond or lake, with supervision, but never on a stream. Supervising adults consult with park personnel, local police, etc., to determine whether the ice is safe for skating.

☐ Girls never ice-skate alone. Girls use the buddy system.

☐ Girls may skate at night if the area is well lit.

Clothing

☐ Clothing allows freedom of movement. Several warm layers are recommended for outdoor skating, including hats and gloves or mittens. Bring a change of socks.

Equipment

☐ Girls receive instruction in selecting the proper skate size. Ice skates are properly fitted, securely laced, and properly tied.

Site

☐ Obtain council guidance in selecting the ice-skating site. Rinks are safest.

Ice Skating Rink

☐ The rink has a smooth skating surface free of papers, candy wrappers, and other debris.

Outdoor Ice Skating

☐ Skating surfaces are checked in advance for thickness, patches of grass, rocks, cracks, etc.

☐ Appropriate rescue and first-aid equipment are on hand (for example, ring buoy, rope, throw bag, pole, ladder, boat).

Emergency Procedures and First Aid

☐ A first-aider, Level 1, is present.

Outdoor Ice Skating

☐ The first-aider is prepared to handle cases of near-drowning and immersion hypothermia.

☐ Basic ice rescue techniques are understood and practiced.

National Organizations

Ice Skating Institute (www.skateisi.com), Professional Skaters Association.

In-Line and Roller Skating and Skateboarding

Planning and Supervision

☐ The rink manager is called in advance to arrange for large groups or for practice sessions. The rink is adequately staffed to monitor the size of the crowd. (Check with the rink manager in advance to learn how many adults, in addition to the rink staff, are needed to supervise the group.)

☐ Leaders supervise from outside the main skating floor.

☐ All girls receive basic instruction in skating skills, including how to fall and get up. Practice sessions are scheduled for beginners.

☐ Girls learn to perform basic skating skills before attempting more advanced skills. Warm-up exercises are done before any strenuous skating; cool-down exercises end the sessions.

☐ Skaters are instructed in safety rules by the leader or rink manager or both.

☐ The rules of the rink are observed. For example:
- Everyone skates in the same direction.

- Girls do not stop in the main skating area.
- Skaters yield the right-of-way to those already in the rink.
- Skaters do not cut across the paths of other skaters.
- Skaters do not push, shove, or skate into others.
- A falling skater does not grab hold of another skater.
- A fallen skater rises quickly, unless injured.

☐ Loose or sharp articles, such as handbags, combs, and keys, are not carried in pockets, hands, hair, or anyplace where they might injure a skater in the event of a fall, fall to the floor, or injure another skater.

☐ Outdoors, girls skate in areas where traffic or pedestrians will not interfere. Check local ordinances for any restrictions. Girls skate in the street or in a parking lot only if it is closed to traffic. When skating on a walkway, yield to pedestrians. Skate on the right side, pass on the left.

☐ Girls do not skate faster than their ability to stop.

☐ Girls use the buddy system.

☐ Skaters are alert to their surroundings. Girls do not wear headphones while skating.

☐ Girls skate at night only in well-lit areas.

Clothing

☐ Clothing allows freedom of movement. Long-sleeved shirts help to prevent scrapes.

Equipment

☐ Girls receive instruction in selecting the proper skate size. Skates are properly fitted, securely laced, and properly tied.

☐ Skate wheels, boots, and plates are kept clean and in good condition and are inspected. Girls never skate with broken or missing laces. No dangling decorations are attached to laces.

☐ When skating outdoors, protective gear includes snug-fitting elbow pads and kneepads, wrist guards that fit like gloves, and a bike helmet or a helmet with the American National Standards Institute or SNELL Memorial Foundation seal or both. Helmets should be as snug as possible and be worn low over the forehead, approximately one inch above the eyebrows.

Site

☐ Council guidance is obtained in selecting the skating site. Rinks are safest.

☐ The rink should have a smooth skating surface free of papers, candy wrappers, and other debris.

☐ Local ordinances or parks offices are checked to see whether skating is permitted on bike paths or in city parks.

☐ Outdoor skating surfaces are checked in advance for cracks, uneven joints and grooves, twigs, pebbles, or bits of glass that might cause a fall.

☐ Avoid water, sand, and debris, which will damage the wheel bearings.

National Organizations

Roller Skating Association International (www.rollerskating.org), International In-Line Skating Association.

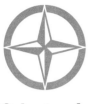

Orienteering

Planning and Supervision

☐ Participants receive instruction from a person experienced in orienteering before navigating an orienteering course. First-timers participate on a beginner-level course. Girls with previous topographic map-reading experience may be eligible to attempt an advanced beginners' course.

☐ Daisy and Brownie Girl Scouts go in small groups with an adult who has had basic instruction in orienteering. They may participate on a String-O course with an adult watching.

☐ Junior Girl Scouts in small groups are accompanied on a course by an adult with basic instruction in orienteering.

☐ Girl Scouts, 11 years of age and older, who have received training may orienteer in groups of at least two.

☐ Competitive Orienteering Courses often require participants to operate independently. While solo competition is not recommended for inexperienced or other program age levels, girls 11 years of age and older whose skill match or exceed the demands of the course may participate in such competitions. As with all orienteering sites, there should be a clear area of safety (Safety Lane), a specific finish time and location and a Search and Rescue procedure designed by the competition's host and the Girl Scout advisor/leader.

Clothing

☐ Girls wear long pants and hiking boots or sneakers.

☐ Girls take proper precautions in areas where poisonous plants or snakes or ticks are prevalent.

Equipment

☐ Each group carries an orienteering map, a compass, an emergency signaling whistle, and a watch.

Site

☐ Whenever possible, girls take part in a meet organized by an orienteering club.

☐ When other areas are used, check for the following:

■ The site selected is a park, camp, or other area with a good trail network.

■ Proper landowner permission is secured to use the site.

■ During hunting season, the orienteering site is in a "no hunting" area with sufficient separation from hunting activity to ensure no accidental contact between hunters and orienteers.

■ Out-of-bounds and dangerous areas are marked on the map.

■ Hazardous obstacles are marked on the ground—they are surrounded by surveyor's tape or a similar marking.

■ The orienteering map is sufficiently accurate so that the participants are not navigationally misled.

Emergency Procedures and First Aid

☐ A first-aider is present at the course finish area.

☐ Each participant is given a specific time limit to complete the course and must check in at the finish area whether or not she completed the course.

☐ Beginning and finishing course times of each participant are carefully noted to ensure that all participants have returned.

National Organization

U.S. Orienteering Federation (www.us.orienteering.org).

Skiing (Cross-Country)

Planning and Supervision

☐ Instruction is given by an adult with experience in teaching and/or supervising cross-country skiing for the age group(s) involved.

☐ The cross-country skiing group has a minimum of four people, including at least two adults. One adult leads and another adult brings up the rear of the group.

☐ Girls get in condition by exercising before skiing.

☐ Cross-country ski area rules are explained and observed:

- Girls ski under control to avoid other skiers and objects.

- Girls yield the right-of-way to those already on the trail. They step to the side to let other skiers pass. A descending skier has the right of way.

- A faster skier indicates her desire to pass by calling "Track, please."

- Girls do not ski close to the edge of an embankment or a cliff.

- Girls do not walk on ski trails.

☐ Sitzmarks (crash craters) are filled in.

☐ Adequate rest stops with opportunities to replenish fluids and to eat high-energy foods are provided.

☐ Girls are trained in winter survival (e.g., snow cave building, white-outs, avalanche avoidance, etc.) as needed.

Clothing

☐ Hats, gloves or mittens, and heavy insulating socks are worn.

☐ A windproof, waterproof jacket is worn.

Equipment

☐ Sunglasses or goggles are worn to protect the eyes from bright glare off the snow.

☐ Each girl carries a water bottle, high-energy food, sunscreen, and lip balm.

Site

At the Trail

☐ The nature of the terrain, potential hazards (e.g., avalanches, frozen lakes), mileage, and approximate cross-country skiing time are known to all group members.

☐ When a latrine is not available, individual cat holes at least 200 feet away from water sources are used to dispose of human waste.

Emergency Procedures and First Aid

☐ First-aider, level 1, is present. First-aider, level 2, is present if planned route is more than five miles from emergency help.

☐ First-aid procedures are reviewed, including those for frostbite, cold exposure, hypothermia, sprains, fractures, and altitude sickness.

☐ The itinerary, with planned departure and return times and names of the cross-country skiers, is left with a contact person. The route is marked on a map. The contact person is advised before the group's departure and upon its return.

☐ Search-and-rescue procedures are written out in advance.

☐ Advance arrangements are made for medical emergencies and evacuation procedures.

National Organization

National Ski Patrol (www.nsp.org).

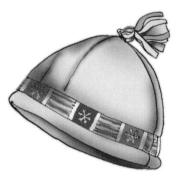

Skiing (Downhill) and Snowboarding

Planning and Supervision

- ☐ Instruction is given by a person with experience teaching and/or supervising downhill skiing/snowboarding for the age group(s) involved.
- ☐ Participants get in condition by exercising before the trip.
- ☐ Participants are taught how to ride area lifts, including line courtesy, loading and unloading, and emergency procedures.
- ☐ Participants ski responsibly. The rules of the ski area are explained and observed.
- ☐ Skiers use the buddy system and use trails and slopes matched to their abilities. At all times, skiers ski under control.
- ☐ Skiers follow these guidelines:
  - ▪ Avoid other skiers.
  - ▪ Avoid objects and obstacles.
  - ▪ Make others aware that they are planning turns.
  - ▪ Do not cross the path of uphill skiers.
  - ▪ Yield the right-of-way to those already on the slope.
  - ▪ Stop on the sides of the slope or trail to rest or adjust equipment.
  - ▪ Move quickly to the side of the trail or slope after falling, unless injured.
  - ▪ Summon the ski patrol if a skier is injured.
  - ▪ Never ski in unmarked or closed areas.
- ☐ There are adequate rest periods with opportunities to replenish fluids and eat high-energy foods.
- ☐ A nutritious, high-energy menu is planned, with beverages provided to prevent dehydration.

Clothing

- ☐ Hats, gloves or mittens, and heavy insulating socks are worn.
- ☐ Windproof, waterproof jacket and pants are worn.

Equipment

- ☐ Sunglasses or goggles are worn to protect the eyes from bright glare off the snow.

Site

At the Slope

- ☐ A meeting place is designated where girls can contact a supervising adult.
- ☐ A list is maintained with the name of each skier and where she will be skiing.
- ☐ There are at least two in each skiing party.
- ☐ The slope chosen is within the ability of each girl in the skiing party.
- ☐ Terrain and potential hazards are known to all the group members.

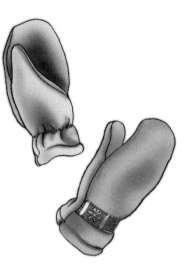

Emergency Procedures and First Aid

- ☐ A first-aider is present.
- ☐ First-aid procedures are reviewed, including those for frostbite, cold exposure, hypothermia, sprains, and fractures.
- ☐ Advance arrangements are made for medical emergencies and evacuation procedures.

National Organization

National Ski Patrol (www.nsp.org)

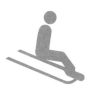

Sledding, Tobogganing, Snow Tubing

Planning and Supervision

☐ Girls receive basic instruction in sledding safety and conduct rules.

☐ Girls learn to perform basic steering skills, including how to slow down.

☐ Conditions are monitored, and breaks are taken to prevent hypothermia and frostbite.

☐ Girls slide downhill feet first to reduce potential for head injuries from collisions.

☐ Girls and leaders agree on the portion of slope to be used for sledding and the portion to be used for walking uphill.

☐ On hills provided for snow tubing, girls review and obey posted rules.

Site

☐ Sledding is conducted in an area free of vehicles.

☐ The site has no obstructions such as rocks, trees, or signposts.

Emergency Procedures and First Aid

☐ A first-aider is present.

Snowshoeing

Planning and Supervision

☐ Instruction is given by an adult with experience in teaching and/or supervising snowshoeing.

☐ The snowshoeing group has a minimum of four people, including at least two adults.

☐ One adult leads and another adult brings up the rear of the group.

☐ Girls get in condition by exercising before snowshoeing.

☐ Girls are instructed in basic snowshoeing techniques. Leaders are aware of each girl's ability. Practice sessions are scheduled for beginners.

☐ Girls are trained in winter survival, such as snow cave building, whiteouts, and avalanche avoidance, as needed.

☐ There are adequate rest stops with opportunities to replenish fluids and eat high-energy foods.

Clothing

☐ Gaiters (for deep, new snow), a hat, a windproof, water-repellent parka, mittens or gloves, and water-repellent boots are worn.

☐ Sunglasses or goggles are worn to protect the eyes from bright glare off the snow.

Equipment

☐ The equipment is appropriate for the type of terrain, the participant's body weight, and the weight of any backpack.

☐ Girls use snowshoes and bindings that fit properly.

☐ One or two ski poles may be used for balance. The pole(s) is the proper size for the girl.

☐ Each girl carries a water bottle, high-energy food, sunscreen, and lip balm.

Site

☐ Terrain and potential hazards (e.g., frozen lakes, avalanches), mileage, and approximate snowshoeing time are known to all group members in advance.

☐ When a latrine is not available, human waste is disposed of at least 200 feet away from water sources. Tampons, sanitary supplies, and toilet paper are packed out.

Emergency Procedures and First Aid

☐ First-aider, level 1, is present. First-aider, level 2, is present if planned route is more than five miles from emergency help.

☐ First-aid procedures are reviewed, including those for frostbite, cold exposure, hypothermia, sprains, fractures, and altitude sickness.

□ Search-and-rescue procedures are written out in advance.

National Organizations
National Ski Patrol (www.nsp.org).

Other Land Sports

Planning and Supervision

□ See the activity checklists under Step 1 on pages 81–83 and under Step 2 for "Land Sports" on page 94.

□ Where necessary, trained officials administer the rules of the sport.

□ Girls do conditioning exercises and practice basic skills.

□ Girls are instructed in the rules of the sport, safety guidelines, expected behaviors, and issues of fair play.

□ Girls do warm-up, cool-down, and stretching exercises to reduce sprains, strains, and other injuries.

□ In competition, girls are matched in age, weight, height, skill, and physical maturity.

□ In team sports, positions and sides are rotated to prevent domination of the game and to allow for full participation.

□ Trained spotters and/or instructors' assistants are used for individual sports such as gymnastics.

□ Practice sessions and games are properly supervised and of reasonable length.

□ Practice or competition occurs only when an instructor and/or supervisor is present at the site of play.

□ Sufficient rest periods are given to avoid overexertion and to replenish fluids.

Clothing
See Step 1 activity checkpoints on pages 81–83 and Step Two activity checkpoints for "Land Sports" on pages 94–95.

Equipment
See Step 1 activity checkpoints on pages 81–83 and Step 2 activity checkpoints for "Land Sports" on pages 94–95.

□ There are sufficient floor mats for gymnastics, tumbling, and similar activities.

□ Girls who wear eyeglasses have shatterproof lenses or wear eyeglass guards. A band should be worn to hold eyeglasses securely.

Site
See Step 1 activity checkpoints on pages 81–83 and Step 2 activity checkpoints for "Land Sports" on pages 94–95.

□ Playing surfaces are smooth and clear of obstructions, broken glass, etc.

□ Playing areas have clearly marked boundaries and adequate space for girls to move around freely.

□ Where necessary, there is adequate protection for spectators.

□ Outdoor activity is suspended during an electrical storm or in very hot, humid weather.

□ Ample drinking water is available.

Emergency Procedures and First-Aid
See Step 1 activity checkpoints on pages 81–83 and Step 2 activity checkpoints for "Land Sports" on pages 94–95.

□ Fatigued or injured girls are removed from competition and cared for promptly.

□ A seriously injured girl is moved by trained rescue personnel. An injured girl is not returned to practice or competition without the written approval of a physician.

National Organizations
American Alliance for Health, Physical Education, Recreation, and Dance (www.aahperd.org); National Association for Girls and Women in Sport (www.aahperd.org/nagws).

CHAPTER 10
Water Activities

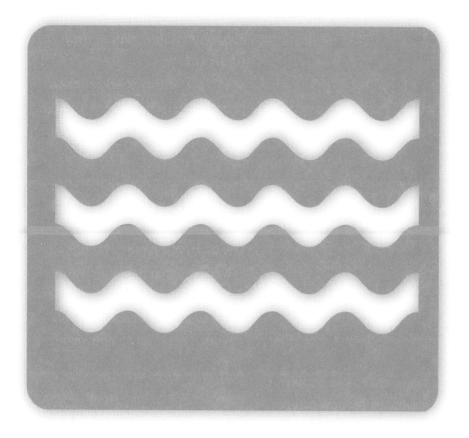

In swimming and small-craft activities, safety is of primary importance. Each girl and adult is accountable for her own behavior and for conducting herself according to waterfront rules, including following instructions, swimming in assigned areas, and watching out for her buddy.

Step 2

Activity Checkpoints

The leader/advisor must review the checkpoints under Step 1 and Step 2 before proceeding to the checkpoints under a specific water activity.

Planning and Supervision

□ Be sure supervising adults have current certification and/or documented experience in specialty areas such as swimming, canoeing, or windsurfing.

□ Determine the number of supervisors for a given aquatic activity by the skill level of the participants, the degree of risk, and environmental conditions.

□ Be sure girls feel safe and confident **in** the water before participating in activities **on** the water. To determine each participant's comfort in the water, conduct a safety exercise such as the following when water temperatures are acceptable: Under the supervision of a certified lifeguard, participants practice putting on a life jacket, entering the water, righting themselves, and coming to the surface. They practice floating and moving with minimal progress.

- Follow the basic leader-to-participant ratios for small-craft activities in Standard 13 on page 69 for events, trips, and group camping. Ratios may be increased, depending on:
  - Number of craft
  - Size of craft
  - Age level of girls
  - Number of girls
  - Experience level of girls
  - Type of activity—instruction, recreation, tripping, etc.
  - Difficulty of activity
  - Size of body of water
  - Wind conditions
  - Tides and currents
  - Flatwater or whitewater
  - Turbidity
  - Bottom conditions
  - Shoreline
  - Proximity of other boats
- Be sure instructions in boating safety and emergency procedures are given and are thoroughly reviewed and practiced while on land, including:
  - Preventing overloading
  - Properly distributing weight
  - Safe boarding and movement on the craft
  - General craft handling
  - "Rules of the road" for water traffic
  - Use of emergency equipment
  - Basic emergency procedures for man overboard, rough weather, firefighting
  - Self-rescue
  - Basic communication systems between craft and land, such as hand signals, whistles, horns, and flags
  - Preventing heat exhaustion or heatstroke
  - Preventing hypothermia
  - Distress signaling
  - Emergency weather procedures, such as in an electrical storm or high winds
  - Towing procedures
- Be sure a system for recalling craft that is both audible and visible is taught.
- Be sure that on a controlled waterfront, a system is in place to determine the location of boaters, such as a checkboard system.
- Make sure craft weight and capacity are not exceeded (some craft have the maximum capacity clearly displayed). Consider weather and water conditions, weight of the passengers, and equipment.

Equipment

- Be sure small craft are seaworthy, fit for water conditions, and used only for designated purposes.
- Be sure boats comply with U.S. Coast Guard regulations and/or state and local codes.
- **Be sure that:**
  - **Each person wears a U.S. Coast Guard-approved personal flotation device (PFD or life jacket) at all times when boating, regardless of swimming ability.**
  - Each wearable PFD (Types I, II, III, V, and Hybrid) is the appropriate size for the person who wears it (within the weight range and chest size marked on the PFD). Each person is instructed in the proper use and fit of the PFD that she is wearing.
  - Every PFD is in serviceable condition and appropriate for the type of waters on which the boat will be used.
  - Each person demonstrates and practices using a PFD, preferably including an in-the-water experience with the PFD to test the fit and amount of flotation it provides.
  - At least one graspable and throwable PFD (Type IV buoyant

113

cushion or ring buoy or equivalent) is immediately available for each group on the water.

- When watercraft are used beyond the immediate waterfront area, PFDs have whistles attached for signaling purposes.

☐ Check that all equipment required by federal, state, and local regulations for the particular craft and waters is aboard, in serviceable condition, and, if appropriate, labeled "U.S. Coast Guard-approved."

☐ Be sure that no gasoline, liquefied petroleum gas, or other type of flammable liquid is used on board with heating, cooking, or lighting appliances.

☐ Carry a repair kit and tools as appropriate.

Transportation

☐ Check that the driver knows the principles and has mastered the challenges of driving a tow vehicle and trailer.

☐ Check that the driver knows and uses the equipment required by law when trailering a boat.

Site

☐ Observe the same general principles when using small-craft sites that are either council-owned or public, loaned or donated facilities:

- Council guidance is obtained in selecting the area.
- The boating area is separate from swimming areas.
- Water conditions are suitable (consider currents, tides, presence of dams, water releases, underwater obstructions, etc.).
- Visibility is good.

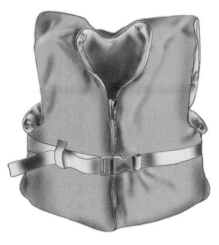

- A lifeboat and rescue equipment are available, where appropriate.

Emergency Procedures and First Aid

☐ Be sure a first-aider is present and a first-aid kit is available.

☐ Be sure to review first-aid procedures, including those for immersion hypothermia, near-drowning, and sunburn.

☐ Be sure a float plan is filed with local authorities and a back-home contact, indicating:

- Names of all persons on board
- Destination

- Description of the craft
- Times of departure and return
- Route to be taken and an alternate route
- Agency or person to be notified if return is delayed
- List of marine communications, if applicable (VHF radio, Channel 16, is constantly monitored for distress calls and is also used as a contact frequency for all recreational boaters)

☐ Be prepared to alter the float plan if weather conditions change.

☐ Teach girls to take shelter away from tall objects in a storm with lightning and thunder. Find the lowest point in an open flat area. Squat low to the ground on the balls of the feet. Have girls place their hands on their knees with their head between them. They should make themselves the smallest target possible and minimize their contact with the ground.

☐ During storms, if shore cannot be reached, secure all loose gear, keep a sharp lookout for other boats and obstructions, head into the wind at a 45° angle, and stay low.

National Organizations

American Red Cross, U.S. Coast Guard (www.usaboating.org), U.S. Power Squadron (www.usps.org).

Canoeing

Planning and Supervision

- **Flatwater canoeing.** One adult is currently certified as a Flatwater, Moving, Paddling, or River Paddling Instructor from the American Canoe Association, is certified in Small Craft Safety from the American Red Cross, has equivalent certification, or has documented experience indicating knowledge and skill in teaching and/or supervision specific to the canoeing activity.

- **Whitewater canoeing.** One adult is currently certified as a Whitewater Instructor from the American Canoe Association, is certified in the Small Craft Safety with Moving Water module from the American Red Cross, has equivalent certification, or has documented experience and skill in teaching and/or supervision specific to the canoeing activity.

- **Tripping—flatwater and whitewater canoeing.** One adult is currently certified as a Moving Water Instructor or White Water Instructor (as needed) from the American Canoe Association, is certified in Small Craft Safety from the American Red Cross, has equivalent certification, or has documented experience and skill in teaching and/or supervision specific to the trip.

- A minimum of two adults supervise any canoeing activity.

- The canoeing skills of the adults are higher than the difficulty of the intended activity or trip.

- The adult instructor/trip leader knows the International Scale of River Difficulty and the Universal River Signals from American Whitewater and its Safety Code.

- The adult instructor/trip leader has firsthand knowledge of the hazards and rapids on the river to be run.

- The river conditions are checked on the day the river is to be run. Participants are taught how to negotiate the hazards and rapids.

- The following instructor/qualified leader-to-participant ratios apply to all forms of canoeing:
  - 1 leader to 12 participants for flatwater
  - 1 leader to 8 participants for whitewater and tripping
  - All forms of canoeing activities conducted on whitewater or semiprotected waters meet the Safety Code of American Whitewater.

Clothing

- For protection against hypothermia, a wetsuit is recommended when the water temperature is below 50°F. When the combined air and water temperature is below 100°F, or when the combination of cool air, wind chill, and evaporative cooling may lead to hypothermia, a wetsuit may be worn.

- Dress in layers—using wool, nylon, or polypropylene pile—under a water-repellent paddling jacket and pants.

- Sneakers or other adequate footwear is worn while paddling.

Equipment

- Canoes 15 feet or shorter hold no more than two persons.

- All persons wear a safety helmet in Class III waters. The safety helmet fits properly and has a flexible, strong, plastic shell with a chin strap and openings for drainage.

- A painter is secured to each end of the canoe. A painter (also called an endline or a grab line) is a strong line that floats and is at least half the length of the canoe.

- Paddles are in good repair and sized to each canoeist. On longer trips or trips involving whitewater, one extra paddle per canoe is carried.

- On trips of 48 hours or less on flatwater, each group carries two or three extra paddles. On longer trips, one extra paddle per canoe is carried.

- For river rescue, all instructors/trip leaders attach a locking blade knife to their PFD or secure it inside the canoe in an easily accessible place. A throw bag is also available.

□ Additional gear (clothing, sleeping, cooking) is stored in waterproof containers or packages and secured in the canoe. **Do not overload the canoe.**

Transportation

□ Canoes are transported on car-top racks or canoe trailers. Canoes are secured with two lines across the top and a line at the bow and the stern.

Site

□ Canoeing is done only on water that has been run and rated. Canoeing is done on whitewater only up to Class III difficulty, as defined by the American Version of the International Scale of River Difficulty.

Emergency Procedures and First Aid

□ A first-aider, level 1, is present for flatwater day trips. A first-aider, level 2, is present for whitewater and overnight trips.

□ A first-aid kit is within the first-aider's reach. The first-aid kit is in a waterproof container secured in the canoe.

□ Take an emergency survival packet—waterproof matches, emergency food supplies, flashlight and extra batteries, a lightweight emergency blanket for retaining body heat, etc.—on all trips.

National Organizations

American Canoe Association (www.acanet.org), American Red Cross, American Whitewater (www.americanwhitewater.org), National Organization for River Sports, United States Canoe Association (usca-canoe.kayak.org).

Fishing

Planning and Supervision

□ Girls are instructed in fishing and use of fishing equipment for minimal impact on the environment and for the safety of themselves and those around them.

□ State and/or federal fishing regulations are followed. Girls and accompanying adults have fishing licenses, where required.

□ One adult watcher certified in American Red Cross Basic Water Rescue or the equivalent is present for fishing from a shoreline or a dock.

□ One adult watcher certified in American Red Cross Basic Water Rescue or the equivalent is present for every 10 girls fishing while wading. More watchers may be needed if the group is spread out or is out of direct sight line.

□ An adult with American Red Cross Small Craft Safety certification or

the equivalent supervises girls fishing from small craft.

□ Fish intended for eating are kept cool to avoid spoilage.

□ Whenever possible, barbless hooks are used and live fish are returned to the water.

□ All fishing gear, bait, and dead fish are removed from the area at the end of the activity.

Clothing

□ Nonslip footwear designed for water sports is worn.

Equipment

□ Girls wading in water more than knee-deep or fishing from small craft wear PFDs.

□ Fishing tackle is appropriate for the size and skill level of the participants and the type of fish to be caught.

□ Tools for removing hooks and cutting lines are available.

□ Basic rescue equipment for reaching assists is available.

Site

□ A site is chosen that avoids steep shorelines, dropoffs, fallen trees, swift currents, submerged objects, and overhead obstructions.

□ Fishing is conducted in an area separate from swimming areas.

Emergency Procedures and First Aid

See page 35.

Kayaking

Planning and Supervision

☐ For river and whitewater kayaking or preparatory classes, one adult must be certified in Small Craft Safety (Kayaking and Moving Water modules) by the American Red Cross, or be currently certified as a Moving Water Kayaking Instructor of the American Canoeing Association, or have documented experience indicating knowledge and skill in kayak rescue and in teaching kayaking skills and/or supervision specific to the kayaking activity being conducted.

☐ For sea kayaking, one adult must be certified in Small Craft Safety (Kayaking Module) by the American Red Cross or have documented experience indicating knowledge and skill in kayak rescue and in teaching kayaking skills and/or in leading trips.

☐ At least two adults supervise any kayaking activity. The skill level of the adults is higher than the difficulty of the intended activity or trip.

☐ The instructor/qualified leader-to-participant ratio is 1 to 5.

☐ For sea kayaking, the trip leader is familiar with water and weather conditions and in tidal areas is aware of tidal fluctuations, currents, and wind patterns that may accompany tide changes.

☐ For whitewater kayaking, the trip leaders are familiar with the International Scale of River Difficulty and with the Universal Signals and the Safety Code of American Whitewater. The trip leader knows firsthand the hazards and rapids on any river to be run.

☐ River conditions are checked on the day the river is to be run. Participants are taught in advance how to negotiate the hazards and rapids.

Clothing

☐ A wetsuit is recommended when the water temperature is below 50°F. A wetsuit should be worn when the combined air and water temperature is less than 100°F or when the combination of cool air, wind chill, and evaporative cooling may lead to hypothermia.

☐ A change of clothes is carried in a waterproof bag secured to the kayak.

☐ Sneakers or other protective footwear is worn while paddling.

Equipment

☐ Each person uses a spray skirt with a release loop.

☐ Each person wears a safety helmet. The safety helmet is properly fitted, flexible, and strong and has a plastic shell with an adjustable chin strap and openings for drainage.

☐ Each kayak is sized for the person using it.

☐ Paddles are sized to the person and the craft.

☐ Each kayak has an adjustable bracing system for the feet and bow and stern grab loops.

☐ Each kayak is outfitted with proper flotation. If used, air bags are checked before trips to ensure that the seals are intact.

☐ For river rescue, each instructor/leader attaches a locking-blade knife, two carabiners, and two prusik loops to her/his PFD or secures them to the kayak in an easily accessible place. (A prusik loop is a mountaineering knot with loops, used with a carabiner for quick tie-offs and z-drag rescues, to recover a kayak pinned against a rock or other obstacle.)

☐ A 50-foot length of tow line (lightweight nylon, polypropylene, or 50- to 100-pound monofilament fishing line) is carried for every three to four kayaks.

☐ Each person has within reach a bailer or a sponge and an emergency survival packet that includes food, clothing, waterproof matches, flashlight and extra batteries, space blanket, hat, and raincoat.

☐ Each person learns and practices appropriate self-rescue and reentry techniques.

- Each person knows cold-water survival techniques and treatment for hypothermia.

- A set of whistle and visual signals is established that allows messages to pass between kayaks.

- Each leader has a compass and a chart of the area.

- Each leader carries a spare paddle, a first-aid kit, a repair kit, and standard safety equipment, including signaling equipment and a paddle float—a solid block of foam or inflatable nylon attached to a paddle that may be used as an outrigger for self-rescue.

Transportation

- Kayaks are carried on car-top rack systems or on trailers designed to haul kayaks.

- Kayaks are secured to the carriers with two lines across the top and lines on the bow and stern.

Site

- Trips are not taken to unknown coastal areas. Locations of all boat channels are known and avoided. Busy channels are not crossed. Surf zones and areas with standing waves are avoided. On long crossings, kayaks are close enough together so that a group decision can be made if wind and water conditions change.

- No trip may be taken on whitewater more difficult than Class III, as defined by the American Version of the International Scale of River Difficulty. Rivers with short stretches of Class IV waters may be run if the girls have the proper skills, are well supervised, and always have the option to carry around the rapids.

Emergency Procedures and First Aid

- A first-aider, level 1, is present for flatwater day trips. First aider, level 2, is present for whitewater and overnight trips.

- A first-aid kit is kept within reach of the first-aider. The kit is in a waterproof container secured in the kayak.

- An emergency survival packet that includes items such as waterproof matches, emergency food supplies, clothing, flashlight and extra batteries, space blanket, hat, and raincoat is taken on all trips.

National Organizations

American Canoe Association (www.acanet.org), American Whitewater (www.americanwhitewater.org), National Organization for River Sports.

Rafting

Planning and Supervision

- A minimum of two adults supervise any rafting activity.

- At least one adult guide with documented experience indicating knowledge and skill in teaching and/or supervising rafting is in each raft to oversee the activity.

- The guides know American Whitewater's International Scale of River Difficulty, Universal River Signals, and Safety Code.

- All rafters are instructed in how to float through rapids, how to breathe while swimming in rapids, and how to swim to shore.

Clothing

- Layers are worn—wool, nylon, or polypropylene pile under a jacket and pants made of coated materials to repel water—to protect the body from getting chilled.

- Laced sneakers or other nonslip footwear designed for water sports is worn on shore and in the raft.

- A wetsuit is worn when the water temperature is below 50°F. A wetsuit is worn when the combined air and water temperature is less than 100°F or when the combination of cool air, wind chill, and evaporative cooling may lead to hypothermia.

Equipment

☐ Each raft is of heavy-duty construction and has at least four air compartments, an adequate number of large D-rings securely attached to the sides, and snug hand lines along the sides.

☐ A safety helmet is worn when rafting in Class III waters. The safety helmet is a properly fitted, flexible, plastic shell with a chin strap and openings for drainage.

☐ Throw lines, throw bags, a repair kit, an emergency kit, knives, whistles, bailers, and a foot pump are carried on the rafting trip.

Site

☐ No trip may be taken on water that has not been run and rated. No trip is taken on whitewater more difficult than Class IV, as defined by the American Version of the International Scale of River Difficulty.

Emergency Procedures and First Aid

☐ A first-aider, level 1, is present for day trips. A first-aider, level 2, is present for longer trips.

☐ A first-aid kit is kept within reach of the first-aider. The kit is in a waterproof container and is secured in the raft.

National Organizations

National Organization for River Sports.

Rowboating

Planning and Supervision

☐ One adult has experience in teaching and/or supervising rowboating or has Small Craft Safety certification from the American Red Cross.

☐ At least two adults supervise any rowboating activity.

☐ On a controlled waterfront, a checkboard system is used to track the number and location of rowboaters.

Clothing

☐ Laced sneakers or other nonslip footwear designed for water sports is worn while rowing.

Equipment

☐ Rowboats have painters (also called end or grab lines) secured to each end of the boat. The bow painter is made of strong line that floats and is approximately the length of the rowboat.

☐ Oars are in good repair and sized and balanced for the rowboat.

☐ A bailer is in each rowboat.

Site

See page 114.

Emergency Procedures and First Aid

See page 114.

National Organization

American Red Cross.

Sailing

The guidelines in this section apply to watercraft up to 26 feet or less in length.

Planning and Supervision

☐ One adult is currently certified as a Sailing Instructor by US Sailing or has Small Craft Safety certification from the American Red Cross or equivalent certification or documented experience and skill in teaching and/or supervising sailing.

☐ At least two adults supervise any sailing activity. The number of supervisors is determined by the skill of the sailors, the degree of risk, and environmental conditions.

☐ Instruction includes launching safety and line handling.

☐ All participants are instructed in the care and use of ropes.

☐ The techniques and skills of the safety position and landing the craft are practiced. Special attention is paid to anchoring in restricted water.

☐ A motorized chase boat is available for all sailing activities, where conditions permit.

☐ Girls are trained in self-rescue procedures in case the wind stops blowing or they are in an emergency situation.

□ Rules set up by US Sailing are followed for sail racing.

Clothing

□ Laced sneakers or other nonslip footwear designed for water sports is worn.

Equipment

□ A repair kit equipped with items such as a screwdriver, pliers, shackles, extra line, a sewing kit, and electrical tape for on-the-water repairs is available.

□ Each sailboat has a paddle as a second means of propulsion.

Site

□ An area for mooring, docking, or landing practice is provided that is away from other aquatic activities.

□ The launching area is clear of overhead power lines.

Emergency Procedures and First Aid

□ A first-aider is present.

□ In a calm-water situation, all participants are taught and practice sailing emergency procedures, such as running aground, man overboard, etc.

National Organizations

American Red Cross, American Sail Training Association (www.tallships.sailtraining.org), US Sailing (www.ussailing.org).

Swimming
Planning and Supervision

Public Facilities

□ Public pools and controlled waterfronts (beaches, lakes, etc.) may be used when lifeguards are on duty. Adults accompanying the group should serve as watchers.

Swimming in Backyard Pools

□ There is one lifeguard for 1 to 10 swimmers. The lifeguard is at least 16 years old and has American Red Cross Lifeguard Training certification or the equivalent. An adult trained in water rescue skills is also present. American Red Cross Basic Water Rescue is recommended for this adult and for watchers.

Swimming Activities in Pools

□ The lifeguard is certified in American Red Cross Lifeguard Training or the equivalent.

Use the chart below to determine ratios.

Swimming Activities in Lakes, Slow-Moving Streams, Rivers, or Oceans

□ One adult lifeguard currently certified in American Red Cross Lifeguard Training plus Waterfront Lifeguarding Module or the equivalent for every 10 swimmers, plus one watcher.

Lifeguard Ratio Planning

□ The ratio of lifeguards and watchers to swimmers may need to be increased depending on:

- Number of girls in one area
- Swimming level and ability
- Girls with disabilities (depending on the types)
- Age level and ability to follow instructions
- Type of swimming activity—instruction, recreation
- Type of swimming area
- Weather and water conditions
- Rescue equipment available

NUMBER OF SWIMMERS	LIFEGUARDS	WATCHERS
1–10	1 adult	1*
11–25	1 adult	2*
26–35	2 persons, at least 1 an adult. Others may be 16 years of age or older.	3*
36–50	2 persons, at least 1 an adult. Others may be 16 years of age or older.	4*

*May be a minor in the state where the activity takes place but cannot be under 16 years of age.

Wading

☐ When girls are wading in water more than knee-deep, an adult with American Red Cross Basic Water Rescue certification or with documented experience in basic water rescue skills is present. A ratio of one watcher to 10 girls is maintained.

For All Swimming Activities

☐ When on duty, lifeguards and watchers are stationed at separate posts and stay out of the water except in emergencies.

☐ Each participant is tested and classified according to her swimming ability. Untested participants are limited to shallow water.

☐ In a controlled waterfront, a checkboard system is used to indicate which girls are in the water and in which swimming area.

☐ In crowded areas, a color system is used for identification. Nonswimmers, novice swimmers, and skilled swimmers each have a wristband or a hair band of a different color.

☐ The length of a swimming period is determined by the swimmer's condition and comfort, weather conditions, and water temperature. Generally, 30-minute swimming periods are sufficient.

☐ Instruction is given in basic swimming rules:

- Girls do not dive into above-ground pools, shallow areas, etc.
- Girls swim in supervised areas only.
- Girls do not swim immediately after eating, when overheated, or when tired.
- Girls swim at a safe distance from any diving board.
- Girls swim with a buddy.
- Girls learn and practice proper use of personal flotation devices (PFDs) and other rescue equipment.

Equipment

☐ Basic rescue equipment is immediately available:

- Reaching pole, approximately 12 feet long (or appropriate to the site)
- Ring buoy or throw bag with firmly attached line approximately 30 feet long
- Rescue tube
- Backboard
- First-aid kit

☐ Electrical appliances such as radios or portable telephones are not used in or near swimming areas.

Site

☐ Whether using council-owned or –operated swimming sites or public, loaned, or donated facilities, the same general principles are observed:

- At public facilities, the water quality passes the local health department tests. Where needed, a copy of the report is obtained from the local health department or a pool test kit is used.
- Bottles, glass, and sharp objects are not allowed in the swimming area or on the beach or pool deck.
- Swimming-ability areas are clearly defined.
- Girls swim only during daylight hours or in a well-lit pool at night.
- Weather and water conditions are suitable for the activity. Wind, waves, water and air temperature, and electrical storms are factors for consideration.
- An emergency telephone is available, whenever possible.

Swimming Pool

☐ Local and state ordinances are observed.

☐ Local health department pool sanitation regulations are observed.

☐ Pool water depths are clearly marked.

☐ Shallow areas are marked "No Diving."

☐ Periodic maintenance checks are made. Maintenance requests and repairs are documented, and records are retained.

☐ Water pH and chlorine are tested and maintained at safe levels. Tests are documented, and records are retained.

121

☐ The pool is adequately filtered so that the water is clear.

☐ The decks around the pool are kept clean and free of clutter.

☐ The surrounding fence and gate or doors to the pool are locked when the pool is unsupervised.

Beach or Other Waterfront Area

☐ Hazards are eliminated or clearly marked.

☐ Girls are instructed to avoid strong currents, sharp dropoffs, quicksand bottoms, rough surf, and other potentially dangerous conditions.

☐ As best as can be determined, the water is free of dangerous marine life.

☐ The bottom is relatively free of debris, sharp stones, and shells.

☐ Swimming, diving, and small-craft areas are separate. They are clearly marked or roped off or both.

Sliding Boards

☐ A watcher signals that the next person may slide when the landing area is clear.

☐ Only one person may be on the slide at a time.

☐ Girls slide in a sitting position, never headfirst.

☐ The landing area is off-limits to other swimmers.

☐ The water in the slide landing area is at least four feet deep.

Diving Areas

☐ The diving area is divided from the swimming area by a buoyed line.

☐ The water in the landing area is a minimum of 10 feet deep for recreational diving boards. The boards are usually 12 to 14 feet long and less than 3 feet above the water's surface.

☐ The water in the landing area is a minimum of 12 feet deep for competitive diving boards. The boards are usually 16 feet long and 3 to 10 feet above the water's surface.

☐ Diving is restricted to water of sufficient depth and checked in advance for submerged obstructions. Diving is prohibited in waters of unknown depth and conditions.

☐ Recreational divers do not manipulate the adjustable fulcrum on springboards. During recreational swimming periods, the adjustable fulcrum is locked in a fixed position, preferably in its most forward position, to reduce the spring of the board.

☐ The maximum water depth extends 10 feet on each side of the center line of the board. If tides, drought, and similar forces affect the water depth, it is checked each time before diving is permitted.

☐ Girls do not dive off the side of the board.

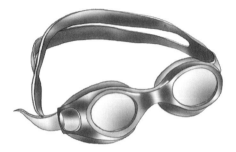

Waterparks

☐ Adults and girls must:

- Read and follow all park rules and the instructions of lifeguards.
- Wear suncreen.
- Drink lots of water to avoid heat dehydration.
- Wear Coast Guard-approved PFDs if they are weak swimmers.
- Know their physical limits. Observe a ride before going on.
- Not dive. Always know the depth of the water before wading in.
- Not run. Most minor injuries at waterparks are caused by slips and falls.
- Use extra care on water slides. They cause a significant number of injuries. See "Sliding Boards."
- In wave pools, stay away from the walls.

Snorkeling

☐ Masks, snorkels, and fins are sized for the individual using them. To function adequately, the mask must fit the face of the user.

☐ Girls learn to swim before going snorkeling. A swimming instructor teaches snorkeling techniques and safety. Girls practice in a pool or a shallow area before venturing elsewhere.

☐ When snorkeling in coastal areas, a PFD is used.

☐ To preserve coral reefs, girls do not stand on reefs, collect organisms, or kick up bottom materials. They do not feed aquatic creatures while snorkeling.

Scuba Diving

☐ Girls who wish to learn to scuba dive must be at least 12 years old and meet the health requirements set by the certifying agency.

☐ Scuba diving is taught and conducted by a scuba instructor certified by one of the following organizations or by a person with equivalent certification:

- Professional Association of Diving Instructors (PADI)
- National Association of Underwater Instructors (NAUI)
- Scuba Schools International (SSI)
- YMCA

☐ Equipment is thoroughly tested and checked by the instructor and the participant before each use.

Emergency Procedures and First Aid

☐ A first-aider is present.

☐ A list of emergency telephone numbers, including ambulance, hospital, police, and fire or rescue unit, is posted.

☐ All girls learn self-help techniques for emergencies, such as cramps.

☐ All girls know and practice basic rescue techniques, such as reaching with a hand or towel, throwing a ring buoy or throw bag, and extending a kickboard.

☐ The procedures to follow in case of a lost swimmer or other emergency are written, reviewed, and practiced.

National Organizations

American Red Cross, National Association of Underwater Instructors (www.naui.org), National Safety Council, Professional Association of Diving Instructors (www.nsc.org), Scuba Schools International (www.ssuisa.com), United States Swimming, Inc., YMCA (www.ymcascuba.org).

Tubing

Planning and Supervision

☐ One adult must be certified in Small Craft Safety, Moving Water module from the American Red Cross, or have experience in teaching and/or supervising tubing activities.

☐ At least two qualified adults supervise any tubing activity.

☐ The experienced adult-to-participant ratio for tubing is 1 to 12.

☐ All participants are instructed before beginning to tube. Girls receive instruction on how to float through rapids, how to breathe while swimming in rapids, and how to swim to shore.

☐ One adult is the lead tuber; another adult is the sweep tuber.

☐ There is only one person to a tube.

☐ Tubes that are tied together are secured very snugly, with no slack between the tubes.

☐ The adult leader knows firsthand the hazards and rapids on any river to be tubed.

Clothing

☐ A wetsuit is recommended when the water temperature is below 65°F.

☐ Laced sneakers or other nonslip footwear designed for water sports is worn.

Equipment

☐ A container with water or juice is tied to each tube to allow each girl to replenish fluids.

Site

☐ No tubing trip is taken on white-water more difficult than Class II, as defined by the American Version of the International Scale of River Difficulty.

☐ No trip may be taken on water that has not been run and rated.

Emergency Procedures and First Aid

☐ A first-aider is present.

☐ A first-aid kit is kept in a water-proof container and secured to a tube.

Water Skiing

Planning and Supervision

☐ All instructors are currently certified by USA Water Ski or have equivalent certification or documented experience, knowledge, and skill in teaching and/or supervising water skiing.

☐ The boat driver has an appropriate license, if applicable, and is skilled in operating the craft, safety and emergency procedures, and managing personnel. USA Water Ski offers a Trained Boat Driver course.

☐ Each boat has a minimum of two adults at all times in all water skiing classes—one to observe the skier(s) and one to drive the boat.

☐ Another adult is on shore, organizing and supervising the girls waiting to ski or watching.

☐ Individuals using the ski boat receive preliminary training in boarding, debarking, self-rescue in capsizing or swamping situations, boat handling for water skiing, trimming, loading, changing positions, using a PFD, and safety procedures for the particular craft.

☐ On a controlled waterfront, there is a system for determining the whereabouts of swimmers and boaters, such as a checkboard system.

☐ The hand and voice signals are posted at the dock area.

☐ Participants know and practice the Water Skier's Safety Code and skier hand and voice signals as defined by USA Water Ski.

Clothing and Equipment

☐ Participants and instructors wear a Type III PFD ski vest while on skis or in the ski boat. Ski belts are not acceptable.

☐ Instructors demonstrate knowledge and skill in operating the boat, motor, and all specialized skiing equipment.

☐ Ski boats are seaworthy, fit the water conditions, have sufficient power to tow a skier(s), are appropriate to the skill levels of the participants, and are used only for the designated purposes.

☐ Ski boats are equipped with a wide-angle rearview mirror.

☐ The ski boat contains at least the following safety equipment:
  - Fire extinguisher
  - First-aid kit
  - Paddle
  - Horn
  - Bailing device
  - Two gas tanks (for outboard motors)
  - Mooring ropes/extra line
  - Boarding ladder
  - Throw bag

☐ Fuel containers are clearly labeled.

☐ Ski lines (tow lines) are at least 75 feet long, in good repair, and of a suitable material.

☐ A single handle is used on the ski line.

☐ Skis are appropriate to the skill and size of the skier.

☐ Skis meet the recommendations of USA Water Ski. Skis are in good condition.

☐ Skis are free of sharp points and edges; ski tips are rounded, not pointed.

☐ Skis have properly sized adjustable foot bindings and are the correct length for the skier's weight and planned skiing speed.

Site

The ski area meets the following description:

☐ A powerboat moving 15 to 25 miles per hour can make a straight-line run of at least a minute, with a broad sweeping turn at each end. With this "dumbbell" pattern, the boat can remain at least 100 feet from shore at all times (state regulations may require a greater distance from shore). Thus, a body of water that is closed to other uses during instruction is at least 2,000 to 2,400 feet long and 250 to 300 feet wide.

☐ There is a designated pickup and dropoff area for skiers.

☐ The ski dock is separate from the swimming area and the sailing dock.

☐ Lifeboat and basic rescue equipment are on hand. Visibility is good (consider time of day, fog, etc.). Water conditions are suitable.

Emergency Procedures and First Aid

☐ A first-aider is present who is prepared to handle cases of near-drowning and immersion hypothermia.

National Organization

USA Water Ski (www.usawaterski.org).

Windsurfing

Planning and Supervision

☐ One adult is currently certified as an instructor by the Windsurfing Instructors of America or has equivalent certification or documented experience indicating knowledge and skill in teaching and/or supervising windsurfing.

☐ At least two adults supervise windsurfing.

☐ The instructor/qualified leader-to-participant ratio is one to four.

☐ All girls pass a basic swimming test to go windsurfing and are able to stay underwater for short periods in order to swim out from beneath the windsurfer if it falls on top of them.

☐ Girls are able to lift a windsurfing rig on land, using proper techniques, before attempting to windsurf in the water.

☐ Girls are trained in self-rescue procedures in case the wind stops or they are in an emergency situation.

Clothing

☐ Girls wear sneakers or windsurfing shoes.

☐ Wetsuits are advised if the water temperature is below 70°F.

Equipment

See page 113.

Site

☐ Windsurfing is taught in a light breeze (1 to 6 knots; 1 to 7 miles per hour).

☐ The wind direction is onshore or sideshore.

☐ The launching area is easily accessible and is clear of overhead powerlines.

Emergency Procedures and First Aid

☐ A first-aider is present.

☐ First-aid procedures are reviewed, including those for cold water-induced hypothermia, near-drowning, and sunburn.

National Organizations

US Sailing (www.ussailing.org), United States Windsurfing Association (www.uswindsurfing.org).

CHAPTER 11
Other Activities

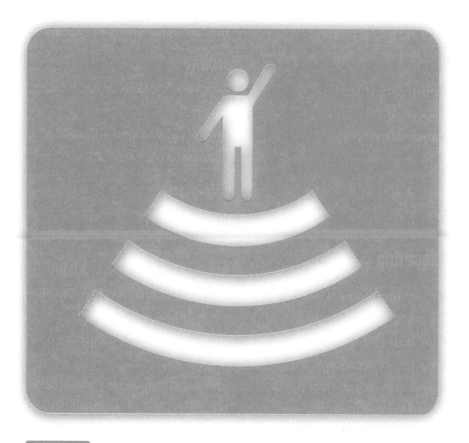

Step 2

Activity Checkpoints

Review the Step 1 activity checkpoints on pages 81–83 before doing these activities. (There are no Step 2 activity checkpoints for this chapter.)

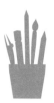

Arts and Crafts

Planning and Supervision

☐ Age-appropriate materials and tools are used. For example, with younger girls, use water-based paints and products that are easily removed from clothes and scissors with blunt ends.

☐ For activities beyond those described in the Girl Scout handbooks and other related materials, the instructor must have documented experience indicating knowledge and skill in teaching arts and crafts.

☐ The instructor teaches girls the basic skills and demonstrates the safe use and care of equipment—for example, cutting tools are used with the blade away from the body.

☐ Activities are appropriate to each girl's age, experience with tools, attention span, and the complexity of the project.

☐ Use of cutting tools, hammers, and spray paints is carefully supervised.

- Supervision is increased when advanced equipment, such as soldering irons, burners, or power saws, is used.
- Kilns are ventilated, and children using them are directly supervised.
- Girls wash their hands after using potentially toxic supplies.

Clothing

- Girls wear appropriate protective clothing, such as gloves for handling hot objects and masks or goggles for protection against sparks, dust, fumes, or debris.
- Long hair is tied back. Girls do not wear loose clothing or jewelry when using machinery or tools with moving parts.

Equipment and Materials

- Art materials are purchased from reputable sources, such as school supply houses. Product labels clearly indicate what the material is and how to write or call the manufacturer.
- **Girls never use donated or discarded material whose ingredients are not known; very old or unlabeled materials may be toxic and are not used.**

- Care is taken to protect children from dyes, pigments, preservatives, and other chemicals that may provoke allergies. Children who are physically or psychologically disabled, or who are on medication, may be at greater risk from toxic materials. **The following materials may be used only after girls have received adequate safety instruction:**
  - Dusts or powders that can be inhaled or that can get in the eyes.
  - Organic solvents, volatile glues, or solvent-containing products such as aerosol sprays.
  - Anything that stains the skin or clothing (or that cannot be washed out of clothing).
  - Acids, alkalis, bleaches, or other irritating or corrosive chemicals.
- Safety tips for handling and storing equipment and supplies:
  - Equipment and supplies are locked in a storage area whenever possible.
  - Safety and operating instructions for dangerous equipment (for example, power tools, kilns) are reviewed and posted.

- Scissors, knives, and other cutting tools are cleaned, oiled, and sharpened, as needed.
- Flammable materials, such as paints and solvents, are labeled and stored in a dry, well-ventilated area out of the reach of young children.
- Equipment and supplies are used for their intended purpose only.
- Turpentine or paint thinner may be used as a paint solvent with adequate ventilation. Gasoline is never used as a paint solvent.
- Solvent- or oil-soaked rags are kept in waste cans that meet fire safety codes and are emptied daily.
- Containers of solvents are covered. They evaporate quickly, and inhalation can be hazardous.
- When girls gather natural materials, conservation principles are taught and practiced.
- Manufacturers' labels on paints, chemicals, and aerosol cans are read before product use. Use these substances in well-ventilated areas only. Do not expose to a flame.
- When transferring substances into other containers, label each container as to content and procedures for use and disposal.

Site

☐ Girls have sufficient space to move around while working; there is space for table work for each girl, when appropriate.

☐ Work sites are well ventilated for activities involving hazardous materials and spray paints (for example, turpentine, spray fixatives, varnishes) or ceramic dust.

☐ Flammable material is used only in work spaces away from ignition sources such as open flames, heaters, and candles.

☐ Provision is made for proper and safe disposal of all waste materials.

☐ Fire exits are clearly marked, and fire safety equipment is on hand.

☐ Food and beverages are not consumed in activity areas.

Emergency Procedures and First Aid

☐ When specialized equipment, power machinery, or chemicals are being used, a first-aider is present.

☐ Emergency procedures are clearly posted for swallowing a chemical, getting a chemical in the eyes, skin contact with a chemical, etc.

National Organization

National Safety Council (www.usc.org).

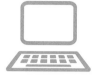

Computers

A group may wish to earn a technology award, e-mail other groups, find information on the Internet, or create its own Web site. GSUSA maintains a Web site, Just for Girls, that provides information about Girl Scouting and invites girls to send their ideas for inclusion on the site. Its address is: www.girlscouts.org/girls.

Planning and Supervision

☐ A consultant with knowledge of computers may be very helpful if group leaders need assistance with these activities.

☐ Find a location that provides group members opportunities to use the computers. See "Site" on page 129.

☐ If girls use the Internet, copy and distribute the "My Online Safety Pledge" on page 130. Discuss online safety issues with the girls, so they know how to conduct themselves safely on the Internet. Monitor the Web sites that girls view. Choose chat rooms carefully, ensuring that they are actively monitored and safe. Discuss the kinds of information girls should not disclose to strangers (full name, address, phone number, e-mail address, photo).

Planning a Web Site

☐ A group that wants to design a Web site must understand that a Web site can be accessed by anyone with a computer connected to the Internet. The Web is an open medium whose sites attract more than just the intended users—including individuals ("cyberstalkers") who prey on children. Such persons search the Web for seemingly innocent details that identify children and the places they go. To protect girls, eliminate personal identifiers from Girl Scout Web sites. Specific information that could jeopardize the safety and security of girls and adults must not be disclosed on a Web site.

☐ To ensure the girls' safety:

■ Use only girls' first names.

■ Never post girls' addresses, phone numbers, or e-mail addresses.

■ Never use pictures of individual girls who are identified in any way without parental permission. (A sample permission form is available at: www.girlscouts.org/girls.)

■ Do not list addresses of group meeting places or dates and times of meetings, events, or trips.

■ Do not allow automatic posting of messages to a Web site by using message boards or guest books that are not continually monitored.

- Ensure that the messaging system does not allow girls and adults to post their e-mail addresses.

Web Site Hyperlinks

☐ Select hyperlinks to other Web sites carefully. The content of potential links should be in keeping with Girl Scout principles and activities. Do not create hyperlinks to Web sites containing paid advertising or selling merchandise to avoid implied Girl Scouting endorsement of the products they offer.

☐ Seek out sites that:
- Enhance girls' participation in Girl Scouting.
- Are tasteful.
- Show diversity.
- Are beneficial to girls, volunteers, and families.
- Are in keeping with the Girl Scout organization's purpose.

☐ Fully explore each Web site link to determine that its content is appropriate to a Girl Scout audience. E-mail the site's Webmaster, requesting permission for the hyperlink. Use similar criteria to determine what sites link to a group Web site.

Group Communication

☐ A group leader who wishes to communicate upcoming events with families of girls should use e-mail instead of posting details on a Web site.

Product Sales

☐ Girls and adults may not post notices on the Internet to sell Girl Scout Cookies or other products from council-sponsored product sales.

Use of Copyrighted Material

☐ A group Web site may not use copyrighted designs, text, graphics, or trademarked symbols without specific permission from the copyright or trademark holder. The basic principle is: If it is not yours, don't use it. Trademarks owned by Girl Scouts of the USA include:
- The trefoil shape
- Daisy Girl Scout Pin
- Brownie Girl Scout Pin
- Girl Scout pins, both contemporary and traditional
- The words Daisy Girl Scout, Brownie Girl Scout, Junior Girl Scout, Cadette Girl Scout, Senior Girl Scout, Girl Scouting, Girl Scouts, and Girl Scout Cookies
- Brownie Girl Scout Try-Its, badges, and interest project awards, their names and symbols

☐ A legal agreement for a "nonexclusive license" to download specific Girl Scout trademarks is available on GSUSA's Web site. It can be found at www.girlscouts.org.

☐ Girl Scout trademarks may be used only in accordance with guidelines for their use. The Girl Scout trefoil, for example, may not be animated or used as wallpaper for a Web site.

☐ Some names (such as commercial products and cartoon characters) are also trademarked and cannot be incorporated into Web site addresses.

Videos and Music

☐ Permission is also required from the author or publisher for Web use of videos and music. This includes posting words to copyrighted songs.

Site

☐ Look for computers available for group use at a library, Girl Scout council program center, school or college computer lab, computer retail store with a training facility, or science museum. Make sure that there are enough computers for each girl to get hands-on experience. (Two girls can share one computer.)

CYBERSPACE SAFETY

Ask each girl to discuss cyberspace safety with a parent, guardian, or adult partner who is doing computer activities with her.

MY ONLINE SAFETY PLEDGE

I will not give out personal information such as my address, telephone number, parents' or guardian's work address/telephone number, or the name and location of my school without the permission of my parents or guardian.

I will tell an adult right away if I come across any information that makes me feel uncomfortable.

I will never agree to get together with someone I "meet" online without first checking with my parents or guardian. If my parents or guardian agree to the meeting, I will arrange it in a public place and bring a parent or guardian along.

I will never send a person my picture or anything else without first checking with my parents or guardian.

I will not respond to any messages that are mean or that in any way make me uncomfortable. It is not my fault if I get a message like that. If I do, I will tell my parents or guardian right away so that they can contact the online service.

I will talk with my parents or guardians so that we can set up rules for going online. We will decide on the time of day that I can be online, the length of time I can be online, and appropriate areas for me to visit. I will not access other areas or break these rules without their permission.

Girl Scout _____ **Date** _____

Parent, Guardian, or Adult Partner _____ **Date** _____

Girl Scout Cookie/Council-Sponsored Product Sale Activities

Daisy Girl Scouts and their parents or guardians may not participate in cookie or other product sale activities.

When Brownie, Junior, and Girl Scouts, 11 years of age or older, participate in cookie or other product sales, review and follow these activity checkpoints.

Planning and Supervision

- ☐ Local ordinances related to involvement of children in money-earning projects are observed.
- ☐ Girls are involved in planning and setting goals for the product sale activity.
- ☐ Each girl's participation is voluntary.
- ☐ Written permission is obtained from a girl's parent or guardian before the girl participates in a council product sale.
- ☐ Girls may use telephones and e-mail to alert friends and relatives to product sales. Girls may not sell products by posting information and making transactions on a Web site on the Internet.
- ☐ A parent, guardian, or other adult must know each girl's whereabouts when she is engaged in product

sales. The buddy system is used.

Clothing

- ☐ Girls wear a membership pin or a uniform or carry a membership card to identify themselves as Girl Scouts.

Order Taking and Selling

- ☐ Girls are familiar with the areas and neighborhoods in which they will sell.
- ☐ Adults accompany Brownie and Junior Girl Scouts.
- ☐ Adults provide supervision and guidance for all age levels.
- ☐ Girls participate in door-to-door sales only during daylight hours, unless accompanied by an adult.
- ☐ When Girl Scouts operate a booth in a store, mall, or other public place, adults must be present at all times.
- ☐ Girls learn and practice personal protection skills as outlined in their handbooks. For example:
  - Use safe pedestrian practices, especially when crossing at busy intersections.
  - Do not enter the home of a stranger.
  - Do not carry large amounts of money. Provision for safeguarding the money is made in advance. Adult support ensures

that girls do not carry large sums of money.

- ☐ The troop leader's/advisor's or other designated telephone number is given for reorders or complaints; a girl does not give her telephone number.
- ☐ When planning sales booths, contact local authorities for permission and for additional safety and security suggestions and assistance.

Emergency Procedures and First Aid

See page 83.

Hayrides

Planning and Supervision

- ☐ Request that the operator supply a certificate of insurance to your Girl Scout council when making reservations.

Transportation

- ☐ Girls do not ride in the hauling vehicle.
- ☐ The driver of the hauling vehicle is licensed to drive a vehicle in the jurisdiction and is at least 21 years of age.
- ☐ The hauled vehicle meets all state and local safety requirements and displays proper identification

showing that these conditions have been met.

☐ The hauled vehicle has protective sides and rear fencing or gates, as well as rear lights in working order.

☐ The hay or straw is properly stacked to prevent slipping.

☐ Sufficient seating space is allowed for each person.

☐ Girls and adults remain seated during the ride.

Site

☐ The hayride takes place on private property at a maximum speed of 10 miles per hour. Public roads and highways are not used.

National Organization

National Safety Council (www.nsc.org).

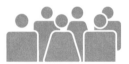

Parades and Large Group Gatherings

Planning and Supervision

☐ Consider the appropriateness of the activity or event, including:

- The needs, interests, and readiness of the girls
- The sponsor
- The needs of the community to be served
- Scheduling concerns
- GSUSA and council guidelines on fund raising, endorsements, collaborating with other organizations, and maintaining nonprofit status

☐ Local regulations and permit procedures are observed for public gatherings, facility use, food handling, certificates of insurance, sales or excise tax, etc.

☐ Instruction is given on safe pedestrian practices, when applicable.

☐ Guidelines for personal protection are observed. Local authorities are contacted for safety and security suggestions and assistance applicable to the parade or event. For safety reasons, name tags or other personal identification is not worn in public places.

☐ Leaders know girls' location at all times.

☐ GSUSA and council guidelines on publicity, photo releases, etc., are observed.

☐ Advance arrangements are made for picking up the girls after the event and parents and girls understand the arrangements.

☐ Leaders and girls pick a place to meet in case of separation from the supervising adult or the group.

Clothing

☐ Girls wear the Girl Scout uniform, pin, or some other means of group identification.

☐ Comfortable shoes are worn for parades and long walks.

Transportation

☐ Adhere to the following points regarding floats:

- Floats drawn by trucks and automobiles are covered by automobile insurance in the name of the vehicle owners.
- Float construction is safe, using no toxic or highly flammable materials, and secured to the body of the float and the vehicle.
- Floats are equipped with portable ABC fire extinguishers.
- Riders on floats have secure seating, or a secure handhold or safety harness if standing.
- Floats are not overcrowded.
- Participants do not walk close to moving floats.
- An adult accompanies girls on any moving float.
- Any coupling of a trailer to a vehicle is appropriate to the load and has a safety chain.
- Nothing is distributed to onlookers from a moving vehicle or a float.

Site

☐ The location for any community event, large group gathering, or parade is inspected in advance, with consideration for the following, as they apply:

- Accessibility to the group and to the public
- Suitability to event size, age groups, and kinds of activities
- Parking availability
- Availability of restrooms

- Security arrangements
- Lighting for evening and indoor events
- Vulnerability to inclement weather
- Proximity to medical facilities
- Availability of police protection
- Fire safety

☐ Occupancy limits are not exceeded for indoor gatherings and events.

☐ Emergency exits are sufficient, well marked, and operational.

☐ Emergency evacuation plan in place.

☐ A food preparation area used for large groups of people meets state and local standards.

☐ Sufficient potable water and restrooms are available to participants.

☐ Provisions are made for garbage removal and site cleanup.

Emergency Procedures and First Aid

☐ There is a designated first-aid station. A first-aider is present. See page 36. A first-aid kit is available.

☐ An emergency vehicle is available at large group gatherings.

☐ Location of the nearest telephone is known at all times.

☐ The leader carries emergency contact telephone numbers.

☐ An evacuation plan is part of written and oral communication with participants for any large indoor or outdoor gathering.

National Organization

National Safety Council (www.nsc.org).

Playgrounds

Did you know? Each year more than 200,000 U.S. children are treated in hospital emergency departments for injuries sustained on playground equipment. Injuries can be reduced by placing resilient surfacing below equipment, better maintaining equipment, improving supervision, and using age-appropriate equipment.

Planning and Supervision

☐ Girls should not use playground equipment without adult supervision.

☐ Leaders teach girls to use equipment properly, safely, and as intended.

☐ Girls should not run, push, or shove on the playground.

☐ Girls should not stand close to a moving swing or other moving apparatus.

☐ Girls wait their turns to use equipment such as slides.

☐ Girls must not tease or play with neighborhood pets.

Clothing

☐ Clothing is snug-fitting or tucked in to avoid snagging or tangling in any of the playground equipment. Wearing clothing with drawstrings on a hood or around the neck is not permitted.

Equipment

☐ Equipment is anchored so that it does not tip, slide, or move in an unintended manner.

☐ All wood parts are smooth and free of splinters.

☐ Wet or damaged equipment is not used.

☐ All metal edges are rolled or have rounded capping.

☐ There are no sharp points, corners, or edges on any components of playground equipment.

☐ There are no accessible pinch, crush, or tearing points on individual pieces of equipment.

☐ Protrusions or projections of playground equipment cannot entangle girls' clothing.

Site

☐ Physical activities are separate from more passive or quiet activities; areas for play equipment, open fields, and sandboxes are in different sections of the playground.

☐ Equipment and activity areas are without visual barriers; there are clear sightlines everywhere on the playground to facilitate supervision.

☐ Traffic patterns are clearly separate for individual pieces of equipment.

☐ Moving equipment, such as swings or merry-go-rounds, is located toward a corner of the playground.

☐ The playground does not have rocks, roots, and other protrusions from the ground that may cause girls to trip.

Surfacing

☐ Hard-surfaced materials, such as asphalt or concrete, are unsuitable under and around playground equipment of any height, unless they serve as a base for a shock-absorbing material, such as a rubber mat. Acceptable playground surfacing materials are rubberlike materials, sand, gravel, and shredded wood products.

Emergency Procedures and First Aid

See page 83.

Science

Planning and Supervision

☐ When any specialized equipment or chemicals are used, an adult with experience and knowledge is present to demonstrate and teach use of the equipment.

☐ An adult is responsible for the safe use and proper care of all equipment and materials.

☐ Science activities taken from the Girl Scout handbooks and related resources should be done as outlined in the materials. The activity should be appropriate for each girl's age, experience, and level of knowledge.

☐ All outdoor science activities, such as field investigations, night hikes, astronomy lessons, cave explorations, or stream studies, are carried out with proper supervision.

Equipment and Materials

☐ The work area is ample and appropriate for the science activity.

☐ When working with any chemical, plant, or animal, the following are observed:

■ Hands do not touch the mouth or face during the activity.

■ Facilities for washing hands and eyes are available at the site.

■ Hands are washed thoroughly after the activity.

■ Equipment is thoroughly cleaned.

■ Used materials are disposed of properly.

■ Chemical substances are used or mixed only when the adult in charge specifically knows the outcome. When chemicals are used, goggles stamped ANSI Z87 on the frame and lens must be worn. Even the simplest experiment can be an eye hazard.

Plants

☐ Accepted practice is not to pick any plant species unless there is a real need. Most observations can be carried out while the plant is in its natural surroundings.

☐ If it is necessary to pick a plant, the adult in charge is familiar with the species and the possible allergic reactions or chemical sensitivity that may be experienced by handling the plant.

☐ Girls wash their hands after handling seeds.

☐ Seeds are not placed in the mouth, as they may be coated with insecticides, fungicides, or other chemicals.

Animals

☐ Whenever animals or objects they use—such as food bowls, water dishes, toys—are handled, hands must be thoroughly washed with soap under running water.

☐ Iguanas, turtles, and other reptiles, as well as pet ducklings and chicks, can harbor the salmonella bacteria, which can be passed on to humans. Contact with these animals should be avoided.

☐ Activities with animals are carried out with sensitivity and concern for the needs of the animals.

☐ Aquariums and terrariums are kept in areas where proper care, temperature regulation, and maintenance are always possible.

☐ Girls are aware of the proper care, feeding, and maintenance of animals and take responsibility for meeting these needs.

Site

☐ There are well-ventilated areas for the use of vaporous materials such as chemicals.

☐ Flammable materials are kept in fireproof containers and in an area away from ignition sources.

☐ Food or beverages are not consumed in an activity area. Hands are washed before eating.

Emergency Procedures and First Aid

See page 83.

National Organizations

Association for Women in Science (www.awis.org), National Safety Council (www.nsc.org), National Science Teachers Association (www.nsta.org).

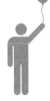

Theme Parks

Planning and Supervision

☐ Obtain full information about the rides and other activities and evaluate them for safety. Discuss with the park manager or safety officer safety procedures, maintenance programs, insurance coverage, and other matters of concern. Verify in advance that the park carries liability insurance.

☐ Each girl is instructed to consider her own personal limitations with regard to rides: how is she affected by height, speed, movement, flashing lights. Theme parks have policies and signs restricting access to certain rides because of height, weight, or other criteria.

☐ Leaders instruct girls to look for and comply with all safety-related signs and instructions given by ride operators.

Clothing

☐ Casual and comfortable clothing suitable for the weather is worn. On sunny or hazy days, protection from the sun is needed.

☐ All hats, glasses, purses, and other such items are secured during the ride or not taken on the ride.

☐ Long, flowing garments and dangling jewelry are not worn.

☐ Girls wear comfortable walking shoes that provide good traction.

Site

☐ Leaders/advisors determine the appropriate time of day and length of the visit to the theme park.

☐ Upon arrival, leaders obtain a copy of the park guide—to facilitate the visit and gain important information on park policies and the location of restrooms and the first-aid station. They pay special attention to any safety tips or warnings and

share this information with the girls.

☐ Leaders/advisors discuss plans for the visit with the girls, and set a place to meet in case of separation from the supervising adult or the group.

☐ In extremely hot weather, girls go on rides and do other outdoor activities in the morning and late afternoon hours, and go inside for meals, stage shows, etc., during the warmest time of the day.

☐ On rides, girls and adults remain seated and always keep their arms and legs inside the car at all times.

☐ Seat belts or restraint bars are always used and are never removed during rides.

☐ Any unsafe conditions, such as slippery floors, broken seat belts, nonfunctioning exit signs, etc., are reported to the nearest park attendant.

Emergency Procedures and First Aid

☐ Check that medical care, first-aid equipment and supplies are available and easily accessible.

☐ In the event of illness or accident, notify the nearest park attendant.

National Organization

International Association of Amusement Parks and Attractions (www.iaapa.org).

Appendix

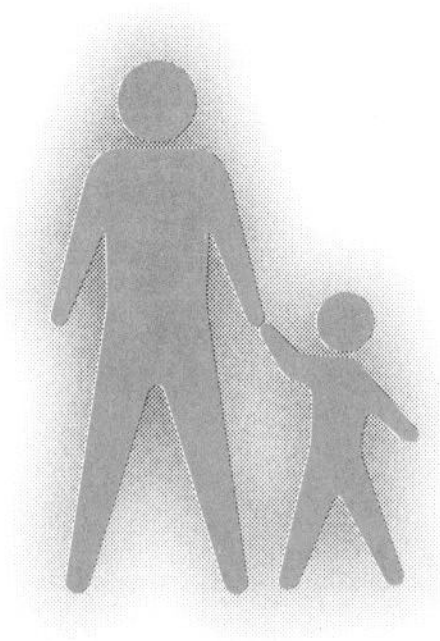

Sample Parent/Guardian Permission Form

Group _____ is planning a _____

Date _____ Time _____

Location _____

Telephone number _____

Arrangements for transportation:

Time and place of departure _____

Time and place of return _____

Mode of transportation _____

Leaders accompanying the girls:

Name(s) _____

_____

Each girl will need:

Equipment and clothing _____

Expenses _____

_____

_____

In case of an emergency, the leader will notify:

Name _____ Telephone number _____

who will immediately notify the parents or guardian.

Leader's signature _____ Telephone number _____

137

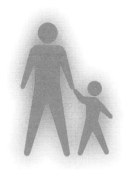

Sample Parent/Guardian Permission Form (page 2)

Return this page to group leader

My daughter, _____ ,

has permission to participate in _____ .

She can participate with reasonable accommodations.

Yes _____ No _____

Please describe: _____

_____

During the activity, I (we) can be reached at:

Address _____ Telephone number _____

If I (we) cannot be reached in the event of an emergency, the following person is authorized to act in my (our) behalf:

Name _____

Address _____ Telephone number _____

Relationship to participant _____

Physician's name _____ Telephone number _____

Additional remarks _____

_____

Parent or guardian's signature _____ Date _____

Sample Letter to a Program Consultant

Dear Consultant:

We are pleased that you have agreed to work with the Girl Scouts as a consultant. We are requesting your services because you have a special interest (expertise, hobby, or skill) that you can share with the girls.

Girl Scouts can gain a great deal working with adults from the community. Of course, not every girl will become an expert in your area of interest, but with your help, each girl will learn more about the world and gain useful skills that may lead her to worthwhile leisure activities or new career choices.

Girl Scouting gives girls from all segments of American life a chance to develop their potential, to make friends, and to become a vital part of their community. It opens up a world of opportunity for girls, working in partnership with adult volunteers.

The Girl Scout program is a continuous adventure. It offers girls a broad range of activities—in science and other academic fields, the arts, the outdoors, sports, and meeting new people—that address both their current interests and their future roles as women. Through activities that stimulate self-discovery, girls grow in skill and self-confidence. They have fun, make friends, and through meaningful community service acquire understanding about themselves and others.

We look forward to your participation in enriching the Girl Scout experience for (describe girls who will benefit—age levels, number, etc.) by (describe requested service of consultant).

I look forward to further discussion with you in the near future.

Sincerely yours,

Signature _____

Typed name _____ Name of council _____

Finding Accessible Meeting Places

When looking at a potential meeting or field trip site, it is important to check all areas; one part may be accessible while another may not. Use the following questions as guides for finding sites that are accessible to everyone. A particular girl, parent or guardian, or other person visiting your group may have other special needs. Add them to the list.

Location

□ Is the site on a route for public transportation?

□ Does one accessible route connect all buildings and facilities on the site?

□ Are there reserved parking spaces for people with disabilities?

□ Are they near the entrance?

□ Are spaces at least 96 inches wide with a 60-inch adjacent access aisle?

□ Are there curb cuts so that people using wheelchairs, carriages, carts, etc., can enter and exit more easily?

□ Are there tactile markings in the sidewalks in front of the curbs to warn people who are blind?

Entrances

□ Is there a ramp at the entrance to the building? Does it go out at least one foot for every inch it goes up?

□ Are all doorknobs to main doors three feet from the ground so that people in wheelchairs can reach them?

□ Have handrails been installed?

Hallways

□ Does the hallway allow at least 32 inches for one wheelchair to pass or 60 inches for two to pass?

□ Is the floor surface smooth enough for wheelchairs to travel comfortably? Is there enough difference in surfaces for people who are blind to get clues?

□ Are door openings at least 32 inches wide?

□ Are door numbers in Braille?

□ If there is an elevator, are floor numbers as well as up/down buttons in Braille? Are all buttons low enough for a person in a wheelchair to reach?

□ Can the water fountains be used by people in wheelchairs or by people with other mobility problems?

□ Are fire alarms low enough to be reached by people in wheelchairs? Are the directions in Braille? Are they equipped with flashing lights so that people with hearing impairments can be warned?

Bathrooms

□ Are bathrooms on an accessible pathway?

□ Are doors at least 32 inches wide?

□ Is there at least one stall with handrails that could be used comfortably by a person in a wheelchair?

□ Do the stall doors swing out at least 90 degrees so that a wheelchair could move in and out freely?

□ Is there at least one counter and sink, and one soap and towel dispenser no higher than 34 inches?

Telephones

□ Is there a clear ground space of at least 30 inches by 48 inches?

□ Is the height from floor to top no more than 48 inches?

□ Are there directions in Braille?

□ Is a TDD (telecommunications device for the deaf) available when needed?

Meeting Rooms

□ How high are the shelves?

□ Are chairs and tables of an appropriate height? Can a wheelchair fit under at least one table, or can one be accommodated easily in an aisle?

□ Do any cabinets or counters stick out into pathways?

□ Can all areas be seen without glare?

□ Have special materials and equipment that will be needed been identified? (Examples: handouts in large print, special pencils, special scissors.)

Procedures for Camping and Other Across-the-Border Visits to Canada of More Than 48 Hours

Together, Girl Scouts of the USA and Girl Guides of Canada have established procedures for camping and across-the-border visits of more than 48 hours. To maintain the goodwill fostered by these exchanges, follow these procedures and complete the accompanying application.

The leader/advisor, at least three months in advance of the proposed trip, notifies the council that the group is planning a trip to Canada and wishes to visit and/or camp with Canadian Girl Guides.

The leader/advisor completes the application, keeps one copy, and sends two copies to the council for approval.

The council, if it approves the trip, keeps one copy of the application and forwards one copy to the Canadian Provincial International Commissioner requesting clearance.

The Canadian Provincial International Commissioner, after negotiation with her areas, writes directly to the leader/advisor indicating what, if any, part of the request can be met and the name and address of the person in Canada with whom the leader/advisor can correspond and plan. A copy of this letter is sent to the council.

From this point on, the negotiations proceed between the leader/advisor and her Canadian contact.

The USA Girl Scout leader/advisor must be sure she has:

◆ Clear directions for the destination of the group (camp, city, home, office, etc.).

◆ The name and telephone number of the person to contact in Canada if plans must be changed or if the group cannot find its destination.

◆ The telephone number of the destination if it is different from the telephone number of the contact person.

Additional Information

It is not possible to arrange for camping at Girl Guide campsites or for contact with Canadian Girl Guides for visits shorter than 48 hours.

Girls and leaders/advisors should bear in mind that at times the numbers of Girl Scouts requesting camping privileges and Guide contacts make it impossible for the Canadian Girl Guides to fulfill every request.

Canadian contacts should not be asked for tourist information. Obtain this by writing the Department of Tourism in the capital of the province where you will be traveling. There

are also Canadian government travel bureaus in some of the major U.S. cities.

Girl Guides of Canada follows similar procedures for across-the-border visits and camping in the U.S.A.

Girl Scouts of the USA/Girl Guides of Canada Application for Camping and Other Across-the-Border Visits of More Than 48 Hours

Council name _____

Council mailing address _____

City _____ State _____ Zip code _____

Group leader's name _____ Group no. _____

Mailing address _____ City _____ State _____ Zip code _____

Trip Plans

Approximate number of girls _____ between the ages of _____ and _____

Approximate number of adults _____ Will be traveling by _____

(Plane, train, public bus, chartered bus, private cars)

We plan to stay the following nights (attach extra sheets if necessary):

	Date	City	Province	Reservation made: name and address of hotel/motel or camp
1st Day				
2nd Day				
3rd Day				

We would like Girl Guides to join us for (check):

daytime activities on _____, evening campfire on _____, overnight stay on _____, and/or we would like to join

Girl Guides if they are having any events on the following dates _____.

We would like to camp on a Canadian Guide campsite in the vicinity of (city and province) _____

from _____ to _____. With a group of Girl Guides? ☐ yes ☐ not necessarily

The following person will know where our group is during each day of our trip and is the emergency contact person:

Name _____ Telephone number _____ Address _____

Group leader's signature _____

Signature of council representative giving approval for trip _____ Date _____

Procedures for International Travel

Leaders/advisors of groups wishing to stay at a world center or a Girl Guide hostel or wishing to obtain a World Association Card of Introduction must follow the procedures listed below.

Stay at a World Center or Girl Guide Hostel

1. One to two years before departure, obtain from your council and complete "Intent to Travel Form A: Request for International Travel Materials." Send to:

Membership and Program Services
　Girl Scouts of the USA
　420 Fifth Avenue
　New York, N.Y. 10018-2798

You will receive an Accommodations Request Form and information about the world center(s) you have specified. For an international preparation packet, contact your council.

2. Six months to two years before departure, as indicated on the form or in the accompanying materials, send the Accommodations Request Form and necessary International Reply Coupons (obtainable from U.S. post offices) to the center or hostel.

3. Upon receipt of confirmations of reservations, send registration fees in the currency requested to the center or hostel.

4. Six to eight weeks before departure, send arrival confirmation (from Accommodations Request Form) to the center or hostel.

Send "Intent to Travel Form B: Request for World Association Card of Introduction" to the council for endorsement and then to Membership and Program Services, GSUSA.

Visit to the Headquarters of a WAGGGS Association

Six to eight weeks before departure, send "Intent to Travel Form B: Request for World Association Card of Introduction" to Membership and Program Services, GSUSA.

A card will not be issued more than three months in advance of departure. Travelers requesting cards less than one month in advance cannot be assured of receiving them prior to departure.

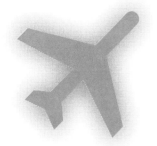

Intent to Travel Form A:
Request for International Travel Materials

Please send an Accommodations Request Form for the four world centers and/or Girl Guide hostels in more than 25 countries (see *Trefoil Round the World* for addresses of hostels)*

Information on world centers

☐ Our Cabaña   ☐ Pax Lodge   ☐ Our Chalet   ☐ Sangam

Name _____

Address _____

City _____ State _____ Zip code _____

Position in Girl Scouting _____

Traveler(s)   ☐ Individual   ☐ Group

Dates of travel _____

Signature of traveler or adult leader of group _____

Council endorsement of individual member and/or group planning to travel:

Council name _____

Signature for council _____

Position _____ Date _____

Mail completed form to:

Membership and Program Services, Girl Scouts of the USA, 420 Fifth Avenue, New York, N.Y. 10018-2798.

* For an international preparation packet, contact your council.

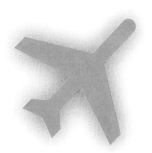

Intent to Travel Form B:
Request for World Association Card of Introduction

Send six to eight weeks before departure. A card will not be issued more than three months in advance of departure. Travelers requesting cards less than one month in advance cannot be assured of receiving them before departure.

Name of traveler or adult leader of group _____

Address _____

City _____ State _____ Zip code _____

Position in Girl Scouting _____

Membership expiration date _____

Countries to be visited _____

Date of departure _____ Date of return _____

Number of adults traveling _____ Number of girls traveling _____

Age range _____

Signature of traveler or adult leader of group _____

Council endorsement of individual member and/or group planning to travel:

Council name _____

Signature for council _____

Position _____ Date _____

Mail completed form to:

Membership and Program Services, Girl Scouts of the USA, 420 Fifth Avenue, New York, N.Y. 10018-2798.

Hotel Security and Safety Tips

Although every reputable hotel works hard to ensure the safety and security of its guests, each guest's cooperation and safety consciousness are still essential. When staying in hotels, leaders/advisors should make sure that every group member knows the following safety and security tips.

In the Hotel

♦ When you enter your hotel sleeping room, always lock the door behind you. Use the chain, if there is one.

♦ If someone knocks at your door, ask who it is before you open the door. Don't hesitate to call the desk to confirm that a hotel staff person is at your door.

♦ Don't call your room number out to a friend while in the hotel lobby or hallways. You don't know who may be listening.

♦ Don't display your key or folder (with your room number on it) at any time, especially in the elevator on the way to your room.

Valuables

♦ Leave all irreplaceable possessions at home. Do not attempt to hide any item in your hotel room. Use the hotel safety deposit boxes, when available. Do not take valu-

able jewelry on a trip! If you do, wear it or carry it with you at all times. Never leave jewelry in your hotel room.

♦ Carry your camera with you at all times.

♦ Never leave cash, traveler's checks, personal checks, or credit/charge cards in your hotel room. Keep a list of traveler's check numbers and credit/charge card numbers.

Luggage

♦ Never leave luggage unattended at the hotel or airport. You may want to lock your suitcase when you leave your hotel room. However, most thieves can open a locked suitcase.

Lost/Missing Items

♦ If you discover something is missing, notify the hotel's security office or the police or both as soon as possible. A list of credit/charge card numbers and traveler's check numbers will help.

Fire Safety

♦ On arrival, carefully read the fire safety information in your hotel room. Be sure to:

♦ Locate the emergency exits on your floor.

♦ Locate the nearest fire alarm and read the instructions.

♦ Keep a small flashlight on your bedside table along with your room key, wallet, and/or passport. A fire can cause the hotel's electrical system to fail.

♦ If adults smoke, be especially careful when smoking in the hotel room. Smoldering cigarettes are a major cause of hotel fires. It is expected that girls will not smoke.

♦ Select a specific place, such as the bedside table, where you will put your room key while in your hotel room. This will enable you to locate the key quickly in an emergency.

♦ In a fire, follow the instructions in the hotel's fire safety information.

♦ If there is a fire alarm or a warning call from the hotel management, do the following:

– Get out as quickly as possible. Don't stop to gather personal belongings. Do take your room key, flashlight, and wallet/passport. Without a key you may be locked out of your room, which may be a safer place to be if the hallways or stairwells are dense with smoke.

– Before leaving the room, feel the door to the corridor. If the door is warm, do not open it. If the door is cool, open it slowly with your foot or shoulder propped against it so you can slam it shut if heavy smoke or flames are visible.

– If the hallway looks safe, go to the nearest emergency exit. If there is smoke in the hallway, first wet a towel and put it over your face to reduce smoke inhalation, and stay low. Close all doors behind you to help block the fire's spread.

– When you reach the emergency exit, feel the door. If it's hot, the fire is in that stairwell, so use an alternate exit.

– Never use the elevators during a fire unless instructed to or accompanied by the fire department. Many elevator controls are heat sensitive and will take you to the floor where the fire is located.

– If your hotel room door is warm or the hallway is dense with smoke, stay in your room and seal spaces around the door with wet towels. Call the hotel operator to report your situation.

– Above all, keep a cool head. The byproducts of fire—smoke, poisonous gases, and panic—cause most fire deaths. Be prepared—and be a survivor.

Additional tips for Hotel Stays

◆ Check with hotel management on security measures to ensure that girls stay in their rooms after bedtime.

◆ Check to ensure that inappropriate videos are not accessible through TVs in girls' rooms.

Lifesaving Awards

Lifesaving awards, a part of the Girl Scout program since the beginning of the Girl Scout movement in the United States, are given to registered Girl Scouts (not adults) who have saved a human life or attempted to save it under circumstances that indicate heroism or risk to their own lives and who have performed heroic acts beyond the degree of maturity and training to be expected at their age.

A Girl Scout, in accordance with the Girl Scout Promise and Law, motto, and slogan, is expected to be resourceful, skilled, and competent—to have presence of mind and to be of service to others. It can be difficult to determine whether an act constitutes unusual bravery and is beyond what is generally expected of a Girl Scout. Each situation is unique, and many factors need to be considered—for example, degree of difficulty of the rescue, amount of assistance received from others, and the circumstances surrounding the incident. A leader who believes that a Girl Scout's action merits a lifesaving award should contact her council for information about the awards and application procedures.

The local council judges whether an act qualifies for a lifesaving award. The council, being close to the specific situation, can gather the facts rapidly, check them for accuracy, and determine whether an act merits a lifesaving award.

Kinds of Awards

The Bronze Cross is given for saving a life or attempting to save a life with risk to the candidate's own life.

The Medal of Honor is given for saving a life or attempting to save a life without risk to the candidate's own life.

When a rescue does not qualify for either of these national awards, the council may give the girl some form of local recognition. The type of recognition awarded should be determined by the nature of the rescue.

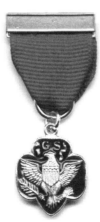

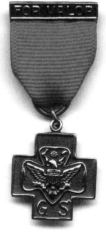

Girl Scout Insignia Chart

The revision of program resources introduced in 2000 presents the perfect opportunity for reviewing the names of official items that girls may wear on their uniforms. While the terminology we are all familiar with, such as "recognitions," served its purpose for many decades, it does not consistently, fully, or clearly communicate the rich and diverse program that Girl Scouts has evolved into at the beginning of this new century.

As a result, GSUSA has developed a systematic way of naming these uniform items that will be clear not only to Girl Scouts but to the community at large. The insignia chart on pages 150–151 illustrates this system and provides examples.

Highlights of the Insignia Chart

1. *Insignia* is the umbrella term used to refer to all official items that girls may wear on the uniform.

2. *Proficiency awards* are insignia from the Girl Scout age-level books that are earned by completing the requirements indicated.

3. *Religious and other awards* are additional insignia that are earned through requirements determined by religious or other organizations or by GSUSA.

4. *Participation patches and pins* are supplementary insignia whose focus is participation, not prescribed requirements. These insignia are developed at the national or council level.

5. *Emblems* are insignia that denote Girl Scout membership at the national, council, and troop levels.

What the Insignia Chart Does

◆ It provides an at-a-glance reference to insignia earned by Girl Scouts at all age levels.

◆ It clearly outlines the difference between one category of insignia and another.

◆ It communicates the richness of opportunities that the contemporary Girl Scout program provides to girls ages 5–17.

How the Insignia Chart Can Be Used

◆ To provide a handy reference tool for new Girl Scout volunteers.

◆ To facilitate the translation of materials into other languages.

◆ To illustrate to potential members, collaborators, and funders the wide range of activities that make up the Girl Scout program.

Note: These insignia are for girls and are listed by the age level at which they are earned.

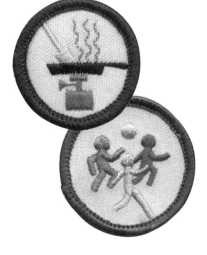

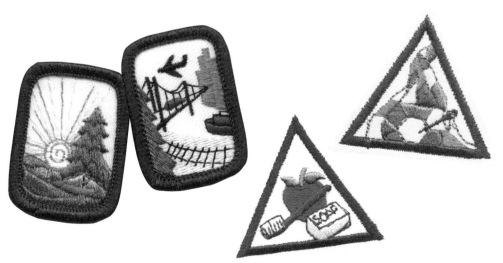

INSIGNIA*
Every Girl Scout item worn on the uniform
(badges, awards, patches, stars, strips, etc.)

EARNED AGE-LEVEL AWARDS

Insignia from Girl Scout age-level books. Earned by completing requirements or by demonstrating understanding of a concept.

DAISY GIRL SCOUTS
- Bridge to Brownie Girl Scouts Award
- Learning Petals
- Promise Center

BROWNIE GIRL SCOUTS
- Bridge to Junior Girl Scouts Award
- Brownie Girl Scout Try-Its
- Girl Scout Cookie Sale Activity Pin
- Our Own Council's Try-It
- Safety Award for Brownie Girl Scouts

JUNIOR GIRL SCOUTS
- Bridge to Girl Scouts 11-14 Award
- Girl Scout Cookie Sale Activity Pin
- Junior Aide Award
- Junior Girl Scout badges
- Junior Girl Scout Leadership Pin
- Junior Girl Scout signs
- Our Own Council's Badge
- Our Own Troop's Badge
- Safety Award for Junior Girl Scouts

GIRL SCOUTS
- Bridge to Girl Scouts 14-17 Award
- Cadette and Senior Girl Scout Interest Project awards
- Cadette Girl Scout Program Aide Award
- Cadette Girl Scout Program Aide Pin
- Cadette Girl Scout Challenge Pin
- Cadette Girl Scout Community Service Bar
- Cadette Girl Scout Leadership Pin
- Community Service Bar in Girl Scouting
- From Dreams to Reality Award
- Girl Scout Cookie Sale Activity Pin
- Girl Scout Silver Award
- Safety Award for Cadette and Senior Girl Scouts

* Check www.girlscouts.org for most recent updates

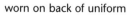

worn on front of uniform

worn on back of uniform

NOTE: These insignia are for girls and are listed by the age level at which they are earned. Girl Scouts have permission to reproduce this chart for Program activity use.

RELIGIOUS AND OTHER AWARDS	PARTICIPATION PATCHES AND PINS	EMBLEMS
Additional awards—earned through requirements determined by religious/other organizations or by GSUSA	Supplementary insignia. Focus is on participation—no set requirements. Developed at national or council level	GSUSA, council, troop membership and identification insignia

SENIOR GIRL SCOUTS
- Apprentice Trainer's Pin
- Cadette and Senior Girl Scout Interest Project awards
- Career Exploration Pin
- Community Service Bar in Girl Scouting
- Counselor-in-Training Award
- Counselor-in-Training Pin
- Counselor-in-Training II Pin
- Girl Scout Cookie Sale Activity Pin
- Girl Scout Gold Award
- Leader-in-Training Award
- Leader-in-Training Pin
- Safety Award for Cadette and Senior Girl Scouts
- Senior Girl Scout Challenge Pin
- Senior Girl Scout Community Service Bar
- Senior Girl Scout Leadership Pin
- Senior Girl Scout Program Aide Award
- Senior Girl Scout Program Aide Pin
- Senior Girl Scout Troop Assistant Pin

Religious and Other Awards
- Girl Scout National Research Pin
- Lifesaving awards: Bronze Cross Medal of Honor
- Various religious awards

Participation Patches and Pins

Examples:
- Building World Citizenship Patch (all age levels)
- Flag Ceremony Patch (all age levels)
- Girl Power patches (Junior and Cadette Girl Scouts)
- Girl Scouting in the School Day patches (all age levels)
- Girl Scouts Against Smoking patches (all age levels)
- *GirlSports* Basics Patch (Daisy and Brownie Girl Scouts)
- Go Global Patch (Brownie and Junior Girl Scouts)
- Investiture Patch (all age levels)
- Learning About Government patches (Brownie through Senior Girl Scouts)
- Patches for both the *Issues for Girl Scouts* and *Contemporary Issues* series (all age levels)
- Project Sew EZ patches (Brownie through Senior Girl Scouts)
- Thinking Day Patch (all age levels)
- Water Drop Patch (Brownie through Senior Girl Scouts)

Emblems
- Brownie Wings
- Council identification strip
- GSUSA identification strip
- Girl Scout Membership Pin
- Membership stars
- Patrol Leader's Cord
- Ten-Year Award
- Troop crest
- Troop numerals
- World Trefoil Pin

Glossary

adult. The age at which one becomes an adult as defined by state statute.

belay. A safety system of ropes and harnesses that is used in challenge courses and climbing to prevent falls.

biodegradable. Anything that can be decomposed by natural biological processes.

buddy system. A safety practice in which two or three girls are grouped to keep watch over each other. In an activity (for example, swimming, hiking), the girls grouped together should be of equal ability.

bungee jumping. Jumping from a structure, such as a bridge, with a bungee cord attached to the body. This is not permitted as a Girl Scout activity.

cat hole. A primitive sanitation method used if a toilet or a latrine is not available; made by scraping away the upper layer of soil, 6 to 8 inches deep, with the heel or a trowel. Cover the waste with soil, and carry out used toilet paper in a plastic bag for proper disposal.

certified. Holds a current (not expired) card, certificate, or other documentation from an established, reputable group, documenting the completion of training in a particular field.

checkboard system. A swimmer's or boater's safety check. Each swimmer or boater has a numbered tag hung on a board. She reverses her tag on the board before going into the water, then turns it over when she returns. The waterfront supervisor then knows exactly how many persons are swimming or boating at a given moment. Sometimes called a "buddy board."

checkpoint. Safety guidelines used in planning and conducting typical Girl Scout activities.

community (service unit) camping event. A group camping event organized and operated by volunteers in a geographic subdivision of the council. The community (service unit) must have council approval to operate the event and must follow the guidelines in *Safety-Wise* and *Safety Management at Girl Scout Sites and Facilities*. Each group is responsible for some of its own plans and scheduling and also participates in activities planned for the entire group. Usually a two- to three-day event.

controlled waterfront. An area where hazards have been eliminated and the water is known to be free of dangerous marine life, debris, and sharp stones and shells. Diving and boating areas are clearly marked or roped off.

core staff. Persons designated by the council to help girls and leaders carry out their specific group camping plans at a given Girl Scout campsite (for example, site director, waterfront staff, naturalist, arts and crafts specialist).

Counselor-in-Training (CIT). A qualified Senior Girl Scout who is taking a Counselor-in-Training course to learn outdoor group leadership skills.

day camping. Camping by the day or camping within a 12-hour program day. Girls from different groups sign up as individual campers and are placed in temporary groups (units). The girls and unit staff plan and carry out activities. Day camping is council-sponsored (requires council approval to operate), and the council provides the staff, facilities, and site.

deadfall. Dry wood, found on the ground, that has fallen off a tree.

diversity. The state of being different. When used to describe people and population groups, diversity encompasses differences in age, gender, race, ethnicity, ability, religion, education, parental status, professional background, marital status, etc.

documented training and experience. Written evidence of competence in a leadership role for a particular activity. This may include records of previous leadership and/or training to instruct the activity, course completion certificates or cards, letters of reference, and/or written evaluation of previous successful leadership work.

drugs. All prescription medications as well as all over-the-counter drugs (e.g., aspirin, cold tablets) that are potentially hazardous if misused.

emergency contact person. The person to call in an emergency or for guidance and advice.

emergency procedures. Basic plans established in advance stating what should be done in case of emergency. Plans should be established orally as well as in writing and should be posted in a highly visible location.

EPA. Environmental Protection Agency.

equivalent training and/or **certification**. Course contents that include all the elements required by a nationally recognized certifying body for that skill.

excursion. A group trip away from a base camp (day or resident) of not longer than two days and one night, planned and carried out by the group and its leader using motorized transportation, with the destination being a particular point of interest.

extended trip. A trip lasting more than three nights (requires a health examination in addition to a health history, council approval, and additional insurance coverage).

fall zone. The surface under and around playground equipment onto which a child falling from or exiting the playground equipment would be expected to land.

first-aider. An adult who has taken Girl Scout council-approved first-aid training from a nationally recognized organization. The level of first aid (level 1 or 2) is determined by the nature of the program/activity. A first-aider must be currently certified and take refresher training as required by the sponsoring organization. The following individuals may serve as first-aiders at level 1 or level 2: physician, physician's assistant, nurse practitioner, registered nurse, licensed practical nurse, paramedic, military medic, and emergency medical technician.

float plan. A detailed itinerary that gives pertinent details for a trip in a watercraft, including departure and return times, total length of time on water, list of persons on craft, where and when stops will be made, and the route to be taken.

frostbite. The freezing of body parts as a result of exposure to extremely low temperatures.

fund-raising. Techniques to appeal to the public to contribute funds to support the program and activities of the organization. Fund-raising often relates to short-term needs and is only part of a fund development plan. Fund-raising is the responsibility of adults.

Giardia lamblia. An organism found in many natural water sources; inges-tion can cause intestinal discomfort, diarrhea, loss of appetite, and dehydration.

Girl Scout camping. An experience that provides a creative, educational opportunity in group living in the outdoors. Its purpose is to use the Girl Scout program, trained leadership, and the resources of natural surroundings to contribute to each camper's mental, physical, social, and spiritual growth.

Girl Scout group. A group of girls and their leaders who meet at scheduled times to conduct Girl Scout program activities. This may be a troop, an interest group, or a unit in a camp setting.

group camping. A camping experience of 24 or more consecutive hours, planned and carried out by a group of Girl Scouts and group leaders, using council-approved sites.

group money earning. Activities planned or carried out by girls and supported by adults, to earn money for the group treasury.

group sponsor. An organization, business, or individual in the community where a Girl Scout group meets that provides funding or a meeting place for the group.

head count. A method of keeping track of the number of participants at a given activity by periodically counting the participants to make sure they are all present.

health examination. A medical checkup given by a licensed physician, physician's assistant, nurse practitioner, or registered nurse within the 24 months preceding a girl's participation in resident camping, in a trip of more than three nights, or in contact sports on an organized competitive basis.

Health examination forms are available from the Girl Scout council office.

health history. An annual updated record of the girl's past and present health status (for example, allergies, chronic illnesses, and injuries) completed by the parent or guardian. A health history is required for participation in physically demanding activities, such as water sports, horseback riding, or skiing. Health history forms are available from the Girl Scout council office.

heat exhaustion. A condition resulting from physical exertion in high temperatures. Symptoms include weakness, nausea, dizziness, and profuse sweating. Also called **heat prostration**.

heatstroke. A life-threatening condition characterized by extremely high body temperature and disturbance of the sweating mechanism.

high-altitude climbing. Mountain climbing that requires use of technical climbing equipment, crossing ice fields, and the possibility of drastic weather changes that can be life threatening. Altitude sickness may occur above 8,000 feet. It is not permitted as a Girl Scout activity.

hypothermia. A life-threatening state of lowered internal body temperature.

itinerary. The planned route of a journey or trip (includes places, dates, and lengths of stay).

kindling point. The temperature at which something will burn.

leader. A registered Girl Scout adult who has received training and who meets regularly with girls to help them achieve the purposes of Girl Scouting.

Leader-in-Training (LIT). A qualified Senior Girl Scout who is taking a Leader-in-Training course to learn leadership skills.

lifeboat, chase boat, or rescue boat. A square-sterned boat equipped with oars, oarlocks, life rings, throw bags, or other life-saving devices; a stocked first-aid kit that includes a single-use pocket face mask; a personal flotation device; and motor and fuel container if allowed by regulation.

lifeguard. A person with current certification in the skills and techniques of lifeguarding from a recognized sponsoring agency and additional training specific to the facility/body of water where she or he will guard. A lifeguard is trained in first aid and cardiopulmonary resuscitation. The type of certification needed depends on the type of facility/body of water where the activity takes place.

minimal-impact camping (low-impact camping). Camping in which no trace of activities is left. The physical landscape of the campsite is preserved as is the solitude and spirit of the wilderness.

outdoor day. A special outdoor event, planned and operated by a council or carried out with council permission and attended by groups or individuals girls. The event may involve one or more groups or may be council-wide or intercouncil.

outdoor education. Use of the Girl Scout program in an outdoor setting to enable girls to grow with regard to each of the four Girl Scout Program Goals.

passengers (on watercraft). Persons other than operator, owner, crew, and employees on board a vessel, except guests on board for pleasure who have not contributed any consideration, directly or indirectly, for their carriage. (U.S. Coast Guard definition.)

passenger vessel. A vessel carrying passengers (see definition above). When in U.S. navigable waters, such a vessel is subject to U.S. Coast Guard inspection and licensing regulations.

patrol. A group no more than eight girls, with a girl leader; usually a subdivision of a Girl Scout group.

personal flotation device (PFD). A life jacket, life preserver, buoyant vest, ring buoy, buoyant cushion, or special-purpose water safety buoyant device designed to keep a person afloat in the water.

pluralism. A system with individuals or groups differing in background, experiences, and culture that allows for the development of a common tradition while preserving each group's right to maintain its cultural heritage. Pluralism is a process involving mutually respectful relationships.

policy. An established course of action that must be followed. The Girl Scout policies are found in the *Blue Book of Basic Documents* and in the accompanying *Leader's Digest*.

portable cookstove. A stove that uses liquid or canister fuel.

preschool age. Children from two to five years of age.

primitive camp (or outpost camp). A portion of a permanent or other campsite where the basic needs for camp operation, such as shelters, water supply systems, and permanent toilet and cooking facilities, are usually not provided.

product sales, council-sponsored. Councilwide sales of authorized, tangible products, such as Girl Scout Cookies or calendars, in which groups may participate.

proficiency awards. Awards earned by Girl Scouts by completing activities in the Girl Scout handbooks.

program consultant. A person who shares her or his interests and special abilities with group members, usually by working directly with girls but sometimes by advising or instructing leaders or camp staff.

Program Goals. The goals of the Girl Scout program.

Program Standard. An established level of quality or achievement for measuring and judging a council's performance in delivering the Girl Scout program to girls.

qualified instructor. An instructor with training and current certification in the activity to be conducted.

rappelling. A means of descending from a vertical cliff, wall, or tower by sliding down a rope. The rope runs through a mechanical breaking device. A safety belay is also used.

resident camping. A camping experience in which the campers live at an established site. Girls from different groups sign up as individual campers and are placed in units (temporary groups). The girls and their counselors or leaders plan activities taking advantage of the resources available at the campsite. The council sponsors resident camping and provides total staff, facilities, and site.

restricted water. A water area that has limited space available for steering—for example, docking and mooring areas.

risk. The possibility of danger, harm, or loss.

safe drinking water. Tap water that the local health department has tested and found safe. All natural water sources are considered potentially contaminated and should be purified before use. Once water has been purified, it should be stored in a clean, covered container. In areas where

Giardia lamblia is present, special precautions must be taken. This protozoan is of increasing concern to backcountry campers. If present in the water source, it can be removed only by boiling the water or pouring it through specially designed filters. Ingestion of *Giardia lamblia* can cause diarrhea, loss of appetite, dehydration, and cramps.

safety belay. A method of stopping the descent of a person on a ropes course that uses an additional climbing rope controlled by a trained belayer.

safety helmet. Protective headgear with a chin strap. Specialized helmets are made for biking, skating, canoeing, and horseback riding and have a seal from an approving authority.

sailing school vessel. A vessel carrying six or more sailing school students or instructors and operated exclusively for sailing instruction (seamanship, oceanography, maritime history, etc.).

sensitive issues. Topics highly personal in nature or rooted in beliefs and values, i.e., AIDS, child abuse, human sexuality, and religion.

small craft. Watercraft under 26 feet long which may include rowboats, canoes, inflatable boats, and sailing craft.

spotter. A person who assists in the execution of physically challenging movements to ensure a girl's safety. Used in activities such as challenge courses, tumbling, and cheerleading.

swimming test. A test that determines a person's ability to handle herself when pitched into the water.

topography. The physical or natural features of the landscape. A topographical map details man-made features, bodies of water, vegetation, and elevation of the landscape.

travel camping. A camping experience carried out by a group of girls who are experienced campers and adult leaders in which the group uses motorized transportation to move from one site to another over a period of three or more nights. Transportation is normally a van, bus, or automobile but may also be an airplane, boat, or train, or a combination of these vehicles.

trip camping. A camping experience planned and carried out by a group of girls who are experienced campers and adult leaders in which the group camps at different sites for three or more nights and travels from one site to another under its own power or by transportation that permits individual guidance—for example, by bicycle, canoe, horse, or sailboat.

trip leader. An adult who accompanies a group on a trip such as camping, backpacking, or canoeing. She or he possesses the knowledge, skills, and experience (e.g., outdoor leadership, trip planning, risk management, first aid, and supervision) required for the trip.

troop camping. *See* **group camping**.

unit. (1) A small group or a group formed at a day or resident camp; campers are assigned to a unit on the basis of age or interest or both for the entire camp session. (2) The portion of a campsite designated as the living and working area for a group or unit of campers.

vehicle. Any device, contrivance, or vessel for carrying or conveying persons or objects.

vessel. A craft for navigation of water; a watercraft.

watcher. A person trained in the use of basic water rescue equipment and procedures who works under the direc-

tion of the lifeguard. American Red Cross Basic Water Rescue certification or equivalent is appropriate.

whitewater. A froth of water containing air, usually associated with rapid currents in narrow or obstructed channels. Whitewater is not dense enough to float a person. A person can easily drown in whitewater.

Types of whitewater are classified in the International Scale of River Difficulty by American Whitewater. If rapids generally fit a classification but the water temperature is below 50°F, or if the trip is an extended one into a wilderness area, the river should be considered one class more difficult than normal.

Class I:

Moving water with a few riffles and small waves. Few or no obstructions.

Class II:

Easy rapids with waves up to three feet wide and clear channels that are obvious without scouting. Some maneuvering is required.

Class III:

Rapids with high, irregular waves often capable of swamping an open canoe. Narrow passages that often require complex maneuvering. May require scouting from above.

Classes IV, V, VI:

Increasingly turbulent rapids that make navigability and rescue difficult or impossible. Classes V and VI are unsuitable for canoes and kayaks.

Index

Membership and Program
8/2000